P9-DVB-869

CARE FOR MAJOR HEALTH PROBLEMS AND POPULATION HEALTH CONCERNS: IMPACTS ON PATIENTS, PROVIDERS AND POLICY

RESEARCH IN THE SOCIOLOGY OF HEALTH CARE

Series Editor: Jennie Jacobs Kronenfeld

Recent Volumes:

CARE FOR MAJOR HEALTH PROBLEMS AND POPULATION HEALTH CONCERNS: IMPACTS ON PATIENTS, PROVIDERS AND POLICY

EDITED BY

JENNIE JACOBS KRONENFELD

*Department of Sociology,
Arizona State University, USA*

JAI

United Kingdom – North America – Japan
India – Malaysia – China

JAI Press is an imprint of Emerald Group Publishing Limited
Howard House, Wagon Lane, Bingley BD16 1WA, UK

First edition 2008

Copyright © 2008 Emerald Group Publishing Limited

Reprints and permission service
Contact: booksandseries@emeraldinsight.com

British Library Cataloguing in Publication Data
A catalogue record for this book is available from the British Library

ISBN: 978-1-84855-160-2
ISSN: 0275-4959 (Series)

Awarded in recognition of
Emerald's production
department's adherence to
quality systems and processes
when preparing scholarly
journals for print

INVESTOR IN PEOPLE

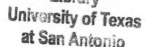

CONTENTS

LIST OF CONTRIBUTORS

Donna B. Barnes	Women's Studies, California State University, East Bay, CA, USA
William P. Brandon	Department of Political Science, University of North Carolina at Charlotte, Charlotte, NC, USA
Patricia Drew	Department of Human Development, California State Universtiy, East Bay, CA, USA
Ashley A. Dunham	Duke Translational Medicine Institute and M.U.R.D.O.C.K. Study, Duke University School of Medicine, Durham, NC; North Carolina Research Campus, Kannapolis, NC, USA
Christine George	Loyola University Chicago, Center for Urban Research and Learning, Chicago, Illinois, USA
Seunghye Hong	School of Social Work, University of Washington, Seattle, WA, USA
Elizabeth Anne Jenner	Gustavus Adolphus College, Saint Peter, MN, USA
Jennie Jacobs Kronenfeld	School of Social and Family Dynamics, Arizona State University, Tempe, AZ, USA
Sally Lindsay	Dalla Lana School of Public Health, Faculty of Medicine, University of Toronto, Toronto, Ontario, Canada

Adina Nack	Department of Sociology, California Lutheran University, Thousand Oaks, CA, USA
Ethel G. Nicdao	Department of Sociology, University of the Pacific, Stockton, CA, USA
Leah Rohlfsen	Department of Sociology, St. Lawrence University, Canton, NY, USA; School of Social and Family Dynamics, Arizona State University, Tempe, AZ, USA
James Rice	Department of Sociology and Anthropology, New Mexico State University, Las Cruces, NM, USA
Teresa L. Scheid	Department of Sociology, University of North Carolina at Charlotte, Charlotte, NC, USA
David T. Takeuchi	Department of Sociology and the School of Social Work, University of Washington, Seattle, WA, USA
Christopher Walker	Loyola University Chicago, Center for Urban Research and Learning, Chicago, Illinois, USA
Dennis P. Watson	Loyola University Chicago, Center for Urban Research and Learning, Chicago, Illinois, USA

SECTION 1:
INTRODUCTION TO ISSUES OF POPULATION HEALTH AND MAJOR HEALTH PROBLEMS

POPULATION HEALTH CONCERNS AND MAJOR HEALTH PROBLEMS: AN INTRODUCTION TO THE TOPIC AND THE VOLUME

Jennie Jacobs Kronenfeld

ABSTRACT

This chapter provides an introduction both to some major issues and concerns in the area of population health and major health problems, especially chronic health problems, and to the overall volume. The topic of population health is reviewed, beginning with the more public health approach of Kindig and that attempt to define the term and the outcomes of interests. The chapter will then move to an examination of the linkages between population health from a more specifically sociological perspective, and especially to relationships between social structure, including socioeconomic status, and health. The last part of this introductory chapter briefly discusses the other sections in the book and each of the chapters within those sections.

Care for Major Health Problems and Population Health Concerns:
Impacts on Patients, Providers and Policy
Research in the Sociology of Health Care, Volume 26, 3–13
Copyright © 2008 by Emerald Group Publishing Limited
All rights of reproduction in any form reserved
ISSN: 0275-4959/doi:10.1016/S0275-4959(08)26001-1

3

INTRODUCTION TO POPULATION HEALTH

In the last few years in medical sociology as well as in public health and health services research literature, a new term of population health has begun to appear. More specifically within sociology, the term population health has been discussed both by demographers as well as by medical sociologists. What people mean by the term has varied, and its application to health problems has also varied. While the specific use of the term "population health" may be relatively new (Kindig, 2007), some of the background considerations of issues related to population health are not so new. Similarly, while population health is being seen as a newer term within medicine, epidemiology, and economics, its sociological roots are longer.

This chapter will first review the essence of the term "population health," relying heavily on the more public health-oriented approach suggested by Kindig. It will then turn to more sociological expositions of population health and how that can be related to relationships between social structure, including socioeconomic status (SES), and health. One definition for population health, provided by Kindig (2007) is that population health "is a conceptual framework for thinking about why some populations are healthier than others." He also states that there is debate about whether population health and public health are identical or different. One aspect of this debate, Kindig argues, is reflected in how journals view their goals and focus. The journal *Milbank Quarterly* redefined its mission to include population health in an explanation by the editor, Gray, that viewed the term public health as having a more narrow focus as a set of activities that are carried out by agencies with official functions in contrast to the term population health as suggesting a broader set of concerns, rather than a specific set of activities (Gray, 2004). With this explanation, *Milbank Quarterly* changed its subtitle from "a journal of public health and health care policy" to "a multidisciplinary journal of population health and health policy." Kindig points out, however, that whether the term population health refers to a concept of health, a field of study of health determinants, or a focus on outcomes, disparities, determinants and risk factors is not yet clear. He also points out that different disciplines that study health services may view similar terms with a slightly different eye. While stating that his article has as goals both identification of areas of agreement across fields and areas in which agreement is not yet resolved, Kindig does focus on four related aspects of population health as an overall term. These areas are: population and health, population health outcomes, determinants of population health outcomes, and policies and interventions (Kindig, 2007;

Kindig & Stoddart, 2003). In discussing each of these, he focuses on population health as having a concentration on the aggregate health of population groups, in contrast to work that has focused, as with intervention research or clinical medicine, on the individual impact. To a sociologist, this sounds very similar to sociological and structural approaches to many topics of inquiry. One expansion in how Kindig views the term is a focus on not only social forces, but also economic forces, biological factors, and environmental factors. An essential issue and focus is measurement of health and health outcomes, leading to the second factor of population health outcomes. Kindig argues this must include both mortality and nonmortality components, preferably combined. Another important linkage here is to the concerns about health inequalities or health disparities.

The last two factors Kindig discusses are determinants of population health outcomes and policies and interventions. He views attention to multiple determinants of health outcomes as crucial to consideration of determinants. He also points out how different fields use slightly different terms, with a strong tradition in epidemiology on focus of risk factors versus more attention to the term of determinants in sociology and economics. A critique within medical sociology that is mentioned by Kindig is that risk factors often refers to behavior and lifestyle factors that focus on the individual and often ignore population level determinants of health. Kindig argues that in population health studies, risk factors that are not part of a causal chain have limited utility. For consideration of the fourth factor, policies and interventions, Kindig argues for a broader consideration of the use of the term policy to include both the narrow conceptualization of the legislative output of the work of elected officials but also codified decisions made in many government and nongovernment settings. The concluding portion of the Kindig (2007) article argues that population health must be defined in the context of the health production function, a heavily economics influenced concept. It is the econometric method that allows for a determination of the independent contribution of each proposed causal factor or determinant (Kindig et al., 2003).

SOCIOLOGICAL DISCUSSIONS OF POPULATION HEALTH AND THE IMPORTANCE OF SOCIAL CLASS

In another recent article, David Mechanic (2007) has also reviewed and discussed the meaning of population health. As a medical sociologist,

Mechanic's approach covers more of the sociological background to this, and also covers a review of the development of the concept. Mechanic points out that "an individualized and medicalized perspective focusing on risk factor identification and intervention" has dominated the last half century (Mechanic, 2007, p. 533). Much of his article reviews in more detail the concept of SES, a core concept in sociology. In more recent years, he argues, there has been a revitalization of a broader perspective that focuses on upstream factors such as social and cultural structures and SES both in the present and also throughout a person's life including in their childhood. In his article, he links population health concerns to a broad area of research within medical sociology that views socioeconomic factors as part of a discussion about fundamental causes of mortality and morbidity.

Link and Phelan began the discussion of fundamental causes in medical sociology (Link & Phelan, 1995, 1996, 2000). They define fundamental causes as including access to resources that will help individuals avoid both a disease and also the negative consequences of that disease. A variety of things linked to SES are part of fundamental causes. This includes money, knowledge and education, helpful social networks, and power and prestige. They also point out that a fundamental cause argument has some focus on contexts. They argue that "the fundamental cause approach asserts that seemingly powerful determinants of health outcomes can be rendered inconsequential when macro level conditions change" (Link & Phelan, 2000, p. 39). They conclude that the association between SES and mortality in many studies has been so persistent because there is a dynamic connection between SES and risk factors. They view their approach as directly antagonistic to claims of modern risk factor epidemiology which argues that if there is full knowledge of intervening risk factors, then more distal social conditions will not be relevant to understand the incidence of disease and death.

Mechanic (2007) adds some very useful implications to the fundamental cause hypothesis by pointing out that advances in biomedical knowledge and technology may increase the health disparities between people of higher and lower SES. If such factors as better knowledge, more money, better social connections, and greater influence to many things in society make it more likely that advantaged people gain access to newer information and services that prevent illness or treat illness, then disparities in health outcomes will occur. An example given in the Mechanic (2007) article to illustrate this point is changing patterns of infant mortality for blacks and whites. Over the past 50 years, infant mortality rates have improved for both blacks and whites, but the percentage of disparity between black and white infant mortality doubled between 1950 and 2004.

Mechanic (2007) rejects two competing interpretations of social class as fundamental. One interpretation is the Barker (1995) hypothesis of fetal and early nutrition. Barker argues that poor nutrition in middle to late gestation and in early life leads to delayed fetal and infant growth and later leads to higher rates of coronary heart disease, high blood pressure, and diabetes. This hypothesis has both strong proponents and strong critics, and while some data from populations and animal studies support the hypothesis, other data from the Chinese famine in the late 1950s and from the famine in Holland during World War II do not support this hypothesis. Randomized controlled trials of maternal dietary supplements in pregnancy have shown only small impacts on birth weight. A second hypothesis is that the key factor underlying the relationship between social class and poor health and mortality is cognitive ability or intelligence. Studies using British data indicate that although cognitive ability attenuates the size of the association between SES and health outcomes, it does not eliminate them. Overall, Mechanic (2007, p. 547) concludes that "the case for cognitive capacity as the crucial factor driving both social class attainment and health remains highly speculative."

Mechanic concludes that education may be the most important SES factor to consider as a fundamental cause of disease and reviews a number of studies examining the link between education and health outcomes. He points out that we need to better understand the linkages between educational pathways and health outcomes. At this point, however, pushes to increase educational levels within US society and in many societies across the world are important both because education is the component of social class most easily modifiable and improved education in people has other socially positive outcomes in addition to impacts on health.

Several recent books by well-known medical sociologists also deal with the issue of social causes of health and disease and health and socio-economic inequalities (Cockerham, 2007; Graham, 2007). Cockerham's book *Social Causes of Health and Disease* argues that some disease is actually caused by social factors. This argument goes beyond the assertion that there is an epidemiological association or a statistical correlation between patterns of illness and social factors. This book represents a critique of an epidemiological approach that treats social factors more as a residual category in analyses that focus more heavily on individualistic approaches. One prime example in the book is smoking. Cockerham argues that the mechanisms of beginning to smoke, continuing to smoke, and quitting smoking are all rooted in social life. The social factors also impact on the experience of illness once the problems are underway. This book also reviews the history of medical sociology and links many of the arguments back to mainstream theoretical concerns in sociology. As with Mechanic who concludes how important SES is and argues for more focus on education, Cockerham also has a strong focus on social class. He views social class as a very important example of the social causes of disease and links this approach also to the fundamental cause argument by arguing that social class qualifies as a fundamental cause because it influences multiple diseases and does so through multiple pathways of risk that then involve access to resources that go on to relate to risks. Cockerham supports his arguments both with American and British data.

A recent British book by Graham (2007) also contributes to these arguments, but more from a British perspective although international data are also used. The book argues that there are causal relationships between unequal social structures such as the labor market and education, social positions such as social class, gender, and ethnicity, lifestyle factors such as diet, exercise, and tobacco use and social inequalities in morbidity and mortality. The first part of this book focuses on defining concepts, the second part on patterns of socioeconomic inequalities across time, place, and disease categories and the third part on causes of health inequalities and policy implications. This book is less theoretical than the Cockerham book, perhaps because it is intended more for readers without a specialist focus, but it also helps to argue the position of the importance of the concept of social class and its linkage to health outcomes.

POPULATION HEALTH CONCERNS AND NEWER RESEARCH ARTICLES

One newer research article to try to present new data on whether SES is a fundamental cause of differences in health status examines data from the Supplemental Security Income (SSI) Program (Herd, Schoeni, & House, 2008). In an introduction to the volume of *The Milbank Quarterly* in which this article appears, the journal's editor, Bradford Gray (2008) points out that the essence of fundamental cause theory is that SES is not just a proxy for other factors that may impact health such as access to health care and health behaviors such as smoking, lack of physical activity, and obesity. Yet evidence from previous studies looking back over past decades has demonstrated that changes in these types of factors have not altered the link between low SES and poor health. Similarly, the mortality shift from infectious to chronic diseases has also not altered this link. A study such as the Herd and colleagues study can add to this debate. The SSI program's purpose is to raise the income of the poorest elderly Americans. Using within-state changes in SSI benefit levels between 1990 and 2000, Herd and colleagues examine the effect of these changes on the states' rates of disability. The article (Herd et al., 2008) links its examination of these issues both to theory and to policy concerns. More generous SSI benefit levels did lead to reductions in disability in the poor elderly. For example, 30% of all single elderly individuals in the study had mobility limitations. An increase of 100 dollars a month in SSI benefits caused the rate of mobility limitations to fall by .46 percentage points. Moreover, they found these findings to be robust when they conducted sensitivity analyses. Medicaid did not confound the effects and the effects also held for married individuals.

In a recent issue of *Health Affairs*, several articles focus on disparities in health, but want to broaden the question to not only focus on the contribution of racial and ethnic disparities to health status and health care, but also to two other key social determinants of health, neighborhoods and education, all in a section on Social Determinants of Health. Acevedo-Garcia and her colleagues (Acevedo-Garcia, Osypuk, McArdie, & Williams, 2008) demonstrate that there are extreme racial/ethnic disparities in children's access to what she calls "opportunity neighborhoods." She argues these disparities come from high levels of residential segregation and that health care policies need to move beyond straight forward health factors to include a consideration of enhancing housing mobility. Gehlert and her colleagues Gehlert, Sohmer, Sacks, Mininger, McClintock, and Olopade (2008) argue that certain social/environmental factors place some groups at a very high risk for negative health outcomes. They create a downward causal model that begins at the population level and ends at disease. They illustrate this approach with mortality disparities from aggressive premenopausal breast cancer. The last two papers in *Health Affairs* in this special section on social determinants of health (Kimbro, Bzostek, Goldman, & German, 2008; Meara, Richards, & David, 2008) both focus on education as a very important factor, as did Mechanic in his discussion of aspects of the fundamental cause approach. Educational disparities in mortality and life expectancy among non-Hispanic blacks and whites in the 1980s and 1990s are the focus of attention for Meara (Meara et al., 2008). They point out that the educational gaps in life expectancy are widening, particularly due to rising differentials for the elderly. In general, recent gains in life expectancy at age 25 have occurred among better education groups, with the exception of black males. About 20% of this differential is explained by differences in smoking related diseases. More recent data from the 2000 through 2006 National Health Interview Survey are the focus for Kimbro and her colleagues (Kimbro et al., 2008). They document the relationship between education and a broad range of health measures, including current smoking, heavy drinking, work limitations, obesity, self-reported health, and low physical activity, looking also at variation by race/ethnicity and nativity. They find interesting variations linked to education, race/ethnicity, and nativity. The foreign born generally fare better across race/ethnicity groups on most of the health outcomes. Much of this is due to more favorable outcomes of the foreign born at the lower end of the education distribution.

These newer papers all raise a number of questions about fundamental causes, education, race/ethnicity, and population health outcomes. Just as these papers reviewed do not cover the complexity and variability of these types of issues, the chapters in the rest of this volume do not exhaust this topic either, but they do make important contributions in a number of areas, discussed in the next section of this introductory chapter.

REVIEW OF THE OTHER SECTIONS AND SELECTIONS IN THIS VOLUME

This volume is divided into five sections. The first section is the introduction to this volume and contains this introductory essay about population health by Kronenfeld. The second section contains three chapters on various chronic disease issues. Each one deals with a different important major health problem: coronary artery disease, arthritis, and obesity. Each chapter uses very different methods and techniques to examine these major chronic health problems in today's world. Lindsay's chapter "How and Why the Motivation and Skill to Self-Manage Coronary Heart Disease Are Socially Unequal" deals with one of the major chronic diseases currently, coronary heart disease. The chapter focuses on the issue of social inequalities, but rather than focusing on the better researched aspect of inequalities in the prevalence of coronary heart disease, the chapter focused upon obstacle to self-management of the problem. The chapter uses a variety of data sources, drawing upon questionnaires, focus group data, and Internet forums. The chapter finds important inequalities linked to gender, marital status, and sociodemographic factors. Another chapter in this section looks at issues of arthritis, another major chronic health problem in the US and other countries currently. Rohlfsen and Kronenfeld use data from the Health and Retirement Survey, a large US survey that is nationally representative of an aging population approaching or in retirement, to examine this issue. Using a variety of social and demographic factors as important control variables, they focus on how different characteristics of arthritis such as severity and duration impact various parts of the disablement process, and look at functional health status, ADLs (activities of daily living) and IADLs (instrumental activities of daily living) as outcome variables. The third chapter in this section by Drew focuses on a different important health problem in the US and developed countries, the issue of obesity. This chapter looks at weight loss surgery patients and is one of the first sociological studies of this group of patients. She uses an Internet-based survey to gather some patient data and then discusses issues of the medical construct of the "ideal patient" and how this links to concerns of patients to obtain the surgery.

The third section of the book looks at two important issues in health for women. In terms of population issues, women represent more than half of the population, and each of these chapters focuses on important issues about gender, illness, and treatment of illness. Nack in her chapter "From the Patient's Point of View: Practitioner Interaction Styles in the Treatment of Women With Chronic STDs" examines how for women with STDs (sexually transmitted diseases), medical encounters occur at a stigmatized crossroads of social control and gendered norms of sexual behavior. The second chapter in this section by Barnes, entitled "I'm Still Here: A 10 Year Follow-up of Women's Experiences Living With HIV" investigates the mothering, reproductive, and living experiences of HIV positive women 10 years after they first participated in a study of their reproductive decisions. The chapter looks at transitions of AIDs from an acute condition to a chronic one and how women in two different locations, California and New York, have dealt with this.

The fourth section of the book includes two chapters on issues related to mental health problems. Mental health concerns are one of the major health problems today. The chapter by Dunham, Scheid, and Brandon explores how primary care physicians deliver mental health treatments for Medicaid patients, and, through a detailed examination of one county, looks at how treatment has changed after HMO (health maintenance organization) enrollment with a mental health carve out. This chapter demonstrates how physicians act as advocates for their clients in the face of both structural and resource constraints on health care. In the second chapter in this section, Nicdao, Hong, and Takeuchi examine the impact of social support and the use of mental health services among Asian Americans. They use data from the National Latino and Asian American Study, a nationally representative survey of the US household population of Latino and Asian Americans, to explore this topic. Looking at this issue in this specialized population, they are able to address issues such the higher use of general medical services among Asian Americans as contrasted with specialty mental health care. They also look at the variations in the levels of social support and use of health services among different Asian subgroups in the population and by nativity status and raise a variety of important issues about the overall low utilization of mental health services by Asian Americans.

The final section of the book includes three diverse chapters that address very important health issues. Watson, Christine, and Walker focuses on a unique population, older homeless people in the city of Chicago. They use both qualitative and quantitative research approaches to examine the severity of health problems in this population and the significant barriers that this population encounters in obtaining health care overall. The last two chapters in this section both deal with issues from a more international perspective. Rice in his chapter "The Urbanization of Poverty and Slum Prevalence: The Impact of the Built Environment on Population-Level Patterns of Social Well-Being in the Less Developed Countries" returns to some of the broader population health themes, in the context of developing countries. The chapter argues that urban slum prevalence is a key factor in shaping population level rates of social well being in developing countries. They examine infant mortality and under five mortality, maternal mortality, and life expectancy at birth. The final chapter in the volume by Jenner, entitled "Shifting Borders of Care: Medical Tourism as a New Dimension in America's Health Care Crisis," looks at the growing trend of medical tourism. This is an understudied area and this chapter uses sociological theory to provide a social analysis of this trend and link it to issues of globalization.

REFERENCES

Acevedo-Garcia, D., Osypuk, T. L., McArdie, N., & Williams, D. R. (2008). Toward a policy-relevant analysis of geographic and racial/ethic disparities in child health. *Health Affairs*, *27*(2), 321–333.

Barker, D. (1995). Fetal origins of coronary heart disease. *British Medical Journal, 311*(6998), 171–174.

Cockerham, W. C. (2007). *Social causes of health and disease.* Cambridge, Great Britain: Polity Press.

Gehlert, S., Sohmer, D., Sacks, T., Mininger, C., McClintock, M., & Olopade, O. (2008). Targeting health disparities: A model linking upstream determinants to downstream interventions. *Health Affairs, 27*(2), 339–349.

Graham, H. (2007). *Unequal lives: Health and socioeconomic inequalities.* Maidenhead, Great Britain: Open University Press.

Gray, B. (2004). In this issue. *The Milbank Quarterly, 82*(1), 3–4.

Gray, B. (2008). In this issue. *The Milbank Quarterly, 86*(1), 1–4.

Herd, P., Schoeni, R. F., & House, J. A. (2008). Upstream solutions: Does the supplemental security income program reduce disability in the elderly? *The Milbank Quarterly, 86*(1), 5–45.

Kimbro, R. T., Bzostek, S., Goldman, N., & German, R. (2008). Race, ethnicity and the education gradient in health. *Health Affairs, 27*(2), 361–372.

Kindig, D. A. (2007). Understanding population health terminology. *The Milbank Quarterly, 85*(1), 139–161.

Kindig, D. A., & Stoddart, G. (2003). What is population health? *American Journal of Public Health, 93*, 366–369.

Kindig, D. A., Day, P., Fox, D., Gibson, M., Knickman, J., Lomas, J., & Stoddart, G. (2003). What new knowledge would help policymakers better balance investments for optimal health outcomes. *Health Services Research, 38*(6), 1923–1938.

Link, B. G., & Phelan, J. C. (1995). Social conditions as fundamental causes of disease. *Journal of Health and Social Behavior, 35*(extra issue), 80–94.

Link, B. G., & Phelan, J. C. (1996). Understanding sociodemographic differences in health: The role of fundamental social causes. *American Journal of Public Health, 86*, 471–473.

Link, B. G., & Phelan, J. C. (2000). Evaluating the fundamental cause explanation for social disparities in health. In: E. B. Chloe, C. Peter & M. F. Allen (Eds), *Handbook of medical sociology* (pp. 33–46). Upper Saddle River, New Jersey: Prentice-Hall.

Meara, E. R., Richards, S., & David, M. C. (2008). The gap gets bigger: Changes in mortality and life expectancy, by education, 1981–2000. *Health Affairs, 27*(2), 350–360.

Mechanic, D. (2007). Population health: Challenges for science and society. *The Milbank Quarterly, 85*(3), 533–559.

SECTION 2:
CHRONIC HEALTH PROBLEMS

HOW AND WHY THE MOTIVATION AND SKILL TO SELF-MANAGE CORONARY HEART DISEASE ARE SOCIALLY UNEQUAL

Sally Lindsay

ABSTRACT

Although much is known about inequalities in the prevalence of CHD, less is known about the barriers experienced in self-managing it. Questionnaires, focus groups, and Internet forums were analyzed to explore obstacles in self-managing CHD. Most people found it difficult and costly to maintain a healthy lifestyle. Gender inequalities included women being more likely to live on their own and with a lower income. Marital status was an issue as several were either caring for an ill spouse or were coping with their recent death. Socio-demographic factors played a key role in influencing people's ability to manage their CHD.

INTRODUCTION

Chronic diseases are now the leading cause of death in developed countries. Over half of Americans live with a chronic disease, placing a tremendous

Care for Major Health Problems and Population Health Concerns:
Impacts on Patients, Providers and Policy
Research in the Sociology of Health Care, Volume 26, 17–39
Copyright © 2008 by Emerald Group Publishing Limited
All rights of reproduction in any form reserved
ISSN: 0275-4959/doi:10.1016/S0275-4959(08)26002-3

economic burden on the health care system. Thus, treating and managing chronic conditions is a key component of health care provision. Evidence suggests that patients cannot rely solely on physicians to improve the management of their disease and therefore, patients need to actively self-manage their illness to maintain their health (Canadian Health Services Research Foundation, 2007). Chronic disease self-management programs developed by Lorig and colleagues at Stanford University have been widely implemented throughout the US, UK, and Australia. Research shows that adherence to such programs can reduce mortality and disabilities, improve quality of life, and reduce health care costs (Taylor & Bury, 2007). A key limitation with these programs is that there have been relatively low levels of participation amongst those who are most in need (Griffiths et al., 2005; Taylor & Bury, 2007; Wilson, Kendall, & Brooks, 2007). Despite this, little is known about the social inequalities and barriers that influence people's ability to self-manage their chronic illness, especially amongst marginalized groups. This is salient because there is a consistently low health status and unequal health burden of chronic disease experienced by those who are older, deprived and from inner city areas.

Examining heart disease is worthwhile because it is the most common cause of death in UK and North America. It is particularly interesting to examine from a sociological perspective because it has a higher social class gradient than in other countries (Peterson, Peto, & Rayner, 2004). Although mortality has been declining, morbidity is increasing. Thus, there is a greater need for patients to self-manage their condition. Heart disease-related mortality and morbidity are particularly prevalent throughout Northwest England, especially within inner cities (Prashar, 2000), where this study is strategically located.

INEQUALITIES IN HEALTH

There is strong and consistent evidence that a higher social class is linked with better health (Curtis, 2003; Prus, 2007). Socio-economic inequalities in health reflect differential social circumstances that are divided along social class. Differences between social class groups in material, cultural, and lifestyle resources influence experiences that can affect differences in health (Prus, 2007). For example, those in higher income brackets tend to have higher life expectancies. Health is also linked with social status where those with a higher job rank have better health, a good standard of living and security. Evidence suggests that the degree of control people have over their life circumstances, especially stressful ones and discretion to act are key influences in health. Thus, having a higher income, social position, and hierarchy can provide a buffer or defence against disease (Curtis, 2003). Those with low incomes often have limited options and poor coping skills for dealing with stress which can increase vulnerability to poor health (Prus, 2007).

The accumulation hypothesis maintains that the health of individuals systematically diverges over the life course where higher social classes tend to experience a less rapid decline in health over the life course (Dannefer, 2003; Prus, 2007; Singh-Manoux, Chandola, & Marmot, 2004). The cumulative effects of leading a healthy lifestyle combined with other advantages in economic and social resources over the life course (for those from a high social class) help to delay morbidity into a shorter period at the end of a person's life. Thus, a person's social position is often linked to the accumulation of future advantage or disadvantage (Schofield, 2007). On the other hand, people from a low social class background tend to experience poor health over the life course. This may be a result of a negative cumulative effect of a poorer lifestyle and fewer resources (both social and economic) (Prus, 2007).

Social inequalities that start early in life are likely a result of unfairness in the social stratification system and are often beyond the control of individuals. Such differences in health can affect immediate health but may also affect the development process and the acquisition of skills that may be useful later in life (D'Arcy, 1998). Indeed, there are significant economic and social costs with pursuing a healthy lifestyle. Material and behaviural aspects of social structure influence inequalities (Townsend & Davidson, 1982).

Inequalities by age, gender, and social class can influence life experiences (e.g., physical, social, and psychological) and can lead to differential access to resources and attitudes (e.g., willingness to take action). Thus, the accumulative nature of life experiences (those in earlier life) can affect responses to health in later life.

The heart patients under examination here are from a deprived area and hence are predisposed to future deprivation and social disadvantage. In Salford, Greater Manchester UK, where this study is located, many wards "suffer from significant problems of deprivation, with low demand and obsolete housing, derelict and underused land and buildings, and poor environmental quality" (Salford City Council, 2005). A health divide is particularly notable between Salford and the rest of England where the life expectancy for men is 2.9 years less than the national average (Salford Primary Care Trust, 2005). Although there have been significant reductions in the death rate from heart disease, the death rate in Salford remains 25% higher than the Northwest average and 50% higher than for England and Wales as a whole (Salford Primary Care Trust, 2005). Thus, examining self-management of heart disease within this area can provide a useful insight into the barriers encountered among those living in deprived areas.

INEQUALITIES IN MANAGING CHRONIC ILLNESS

Evidence suggests that several key barriers exist in self-managing chronic conditions. Such obstacles include physical limitations, lack of knowledge, financial constraints, lack of social support, multiple health chronic conditions, and access problems (Bayliss, Steiner, Fernald, Crane, & Main, 2003; Bell & Orpin, 2006; Bentley, 2003; Jerant, von Friederichs-Fitzwater, & Moore, 2006; Ljung, Peterson, Hallqvist, Heimerson, & Diderichsen, 2005; Nagelkerk, Reick, & Meengs, 2006). Less attention has been paid to inequalities based on social status.

Socio-economic status can have a profound influence on ability to manage chronic illness. People with a low income often lack the resources to maintain a healthy lifestyle. For example, King, Thomlinson, Sanguins, and LeBlanc (2006) found that having a low income posed challenges to patients especially with purchasing medication and maintaining a healthy diet. Although the NHS (National Health Service) provides a rather generous universal service based on clinical need, and not ability to pay, many health goods and services that consumers consider essential are not covered. Indeed, the "accessibility and availability of services has been patchy, posing a particularly severe hurdle for the disadvantaged and vulnerable groups in society" (Sihota, 2003, p. 3). Although the NHS works well for many people, it is often those who are most in need who are the least likely to receive the services they require. For example, in the UK there tends to be fewer GPs (general practitioners) in disadvantaged areas so access to health care can be a problem. Furthermore, the death rate for CHD (coronary heart disease) is 3 times higher in Manchester compared to more affluent areas, yet heart surgery rates are much lower (Sihota, 2003). Examining the barriers experienced in chronic disease self-management among deprived populations is salient because they typically experience a greater burden of chronic illness-related morbidity and mortality (Greene & Yedida, 2005).

Upon looking at gender differences women are more likely to be older than men at the first onset of CHD, which may help explain why they have higher rates of morbidity and mortality after a heart attack (British Heart Foundation, 2005). Women have more undetected or "silent" heart attacks than men, which may result from gender biases in the diagnosis of CHD (McKinlay, 1996). Actual physical differences in CHD-related morbidity are difficult to examine because until recently, women have not been sufficiently included in clinical trials. Even more concerning is that some tests, such as the angina diagnostic test, were designed using a male-only population (Richards, McConnachie, Morrison, Murray, & Watt, 2000). Thus, conventional rehabilitation programs often do not meet the needs of women recovering from cardiac events. Although much is known about gender differences in diagnosis and treatment for heart disease, little is known about gender inequalities in how heart disease is self-managed. Gender is worthy of examination because it influences people's beliefs about health and lifestyle that are associated with disease management.

Marital status and living arrangements also have an influence on chronic illness self-management. Those who are married are more likely to have a better health-related quality of life compared to those who are single (Christian, Cheema, Smith, & Mosca, 2007). Meanwhile, those who live on their own are more likely to report a negative perception of their health and have higher distress compared to those who are married (Soubhi, Fortin, & Hudon, 2006). For example, Bell and Orpin (2006) found that low levels of participation in self-management by those who were single compared to those living in families. This could be a result of single people having less social support; however, the exact mechanism of this relationship remains unclear. There is a need to examine more closely the influence of living arrangements and the moderating effect of gender on these associations (Soubhi et al., 2006).

Age is another factor that is often overlooked in terms of barriers in managing chronic illness. Those who are older are more likely to contend with multiple chronic illnesses (Elzen, Slaets, Snijders, & Steverink, 2007) and may require more assistance to self-manage their conditions because they often have limited mobility and are more likely to live on their own. For example, Beckman, Bernsten, Parker, Thorslund, and Fastbom (2005) found that older people have a difficult time opening bottles, especially women and those with arthritis. Evaluations of chronic disease self-management courses also suggest that younger patients often benefit more than older patients (Nolte, Elsworth, Sinclair, Osborne, & Richard, 2007). Thus, it is important to develop a better understanding of the barriers that aging persons encounter while self-managing their heart disease.

Evidence also suggests that geographic location influences self-management of health. For instance, those with transportation problems and/or those who lack access to self-help groups are often at a disadvantage to managing their health (Bayliss et al., 2003; Jerant et al., 2006). Such barriers particularly affect people in the lower socio-economic strata who experience disparities in health care including reduced access to self-management resources (Fiscella, Franks, Gold, & Clancy, 2000; Jerant et al., 2006; Pincus, Esther, DeWalt, & Callahan, 1998). Those in rural areas may encounter even more difficulties. For example, Winters, Cudney, Sullivan, and Thuesen (2006) found that the rural context influenced the ability of women to self-manage their chronic conditions because they lacked access to health resources. Less is known about the barriers experienced in deprived inner city areas.

Elderly people who live in deprived areas may encounter challenges in making decisions about their health, yet little is known about the specific obstacles they may experience (Lindsay, 2007; Lindsay, Smith, Bell, & Bellaby, 2007). Previous studies that have examined barriers in managing illness tend to focus on middle-class samples while less is known about patients from more deprived areas. Further, most research has focused on diabetes or arthritis while relatively little is known about the inequalities encountered in self-managing heart disease. This study adds to the sociology of health literature by providing an examination of social inequalities within the self-management of heart disease.

METHODS

This chapter draws on a larger project (see Lindsay, Bellaby, Smith, & Baker, 2008) with a sample of men and women ($n = 108$) aged 50–74 from GP's CHD registries. Our sample was drawn from Salford, Greater Manchester, UK because nearly half of the electoral wards are in the top 10% of the most multiply deprived wards in England, including for increased risk for heart disease (British Heart Foundation, 2005).

The focus of the larger project was to assess the influence of a health portal (*heartsofsalford.net*) on the self-management of heart conditions. For this chapter however, the focus is on the barriers and inequalities that patients experienced in managing their heart conditions. Questionnaires from each participant, 30 focus groups, discussion forums, and Internet log data were collected from May 2006 to September 2007. The study received ethics approval from a University research ethics committee and governance clearance from the local Primary Care Trust. The focus groups and discussion forums were tape-recorded and later transcribed verbatim. They were then sorted, coded, and categorized with the aid of NVIVO, a qualitative data analysis program (Richards, 1999). This program assisted in condensing the data and identifying relationships among central themes of barriers and inequalities in managing illness. The project drew on interpretive traditions within qualitative research, where researchers sought an in-depth understanding of the participants' experiences (Green & Thorogood, 2004). The analysis began by reading through each transcript several times and noting emerging themes and patterns. Analysis gradually evolved into the stage of axial coding, which was concerned with the properties of the themes and their inter-relationships.

Table 1 outlines the characteristics of the sample. The age ranged from 50 to 74 with the average age of the sample being 62.9 years. The majority of the sample was male (66.7%). In England, the prevalence of CHD is 7.4% for men and 4.5% in women (British Heart Foundation, 2005). A higher proportion of women (42.9%) had less than a high school education. For the men in this sample, 26.4% of them had less than a high school education, which is likely a result of most of them taking up manual jobs at a young age. The majority of the sample left school at age 16 or younger. A significantly higher proportion of men were married (70.8%) compared to women (28.6%). The majority of the sample [both men (50.7%) and women (71.4%)] were retired. A slightly higher proportion of men (33.8%) were on sickness leave compared to women (14.3%). In terms of self-rated health, most of the sample reported their health to be either "fair," "good," or "poor" with fewer people reporting it as "excellent" or "very good." The majority of both men and women had more than one chronic health problem. The median household income for women was £5,201–7,800 (approximately $10,000–15,000 US); while for men it was £7,801–13,000 (approximately $15,000–26,000 US). Respondents lived in deprived areas of Salford for an average of 31 years.

RESULTS

These elderly heart patients from a deprived, inner city area encountered many barriers and inequalities with regard to managing their health. First, social class had a profound influence on people's ability to lead a healthy lifestyle and often worsened inequalities experienced in other areas. Second, most of them experienced barriers as a result of their age (such as multiple

Table 1. Sample Characteristics ($n = 108$).

	Male (71)		Female (35)	
	Age (avg) $= 62.43$		Age (avg) $= 63.91$	
	n	%	n	%
Marital status*				
Married	51	70.8	10	28.6
Separated	1	1.4	1	2.9
Divorced	10	13.9	10	28.6
Widowed	7	9.7	10	28.6
Single	3	4.2	4	11.4
Education				
Less than high school	19	26.4	15	42.9
High school (Diploma)	14	19.4	10	28.5
Some college	17	23.6	1	2.9
College	10	13.9	4	11.4
University degree	9	12.5	2	5.7
Employment status				
Currently in paid work	11	15.4	5	14.3
Sickness leave	24	33.8	5	14.3
Retired	36	50.7	25	71.4
Self-rated health				
Excellent	5	6.9	0	0
Very good	10	13.9	5	14.3
Good	22	30.6	9	25.7
Fair	22	30.6	15	42.9
Poor	13	18.1	6	17.1
Other chronic health problems	46	63.9	22	62.9
Total household income				
Under £5,200	11	17.2	4	12.5
£5,201–7,800	9	14.1	12	37.5
£7,801–13,000	21	32.8	10	31.3
£13,001–20,800	10	15.6	4	12.5
£20,801–31,200	0	0	0	0
£31,201–46,800	9	14.1	1	3.1
£46,801+	4	6.3	1	3.1

*$p < .01$. *Note:* Sample size varies because of missing data.

health problems and troubles remembering medication). Third, gender also influenced how people managed their CHD where women often encountered more inequalities. Finally, marital status was also salient to many of the participants as several of them were either caring for an ill spouse or dealing with their recent death. The results suggest that socio-demographic factors influence people's ability and motivation to manage their health.

Economic Barriers and Inequalities

One of the key limitations that these patients encountered in managing illness was not having enough material resources, which was largely a result of them being from a deprived, inner city area. Many of them encountered financial difficulties that influenced how they managed their illness. For example many people often found prescription charges too expensive.

> I think one problem with heart disease is that we are always being told that prevention is king but many people on low incomes or with young families find the present prescription costs too high. For example, a parent faced with the choice, would spend money on needed new shoes for their child than on statins for themselves. (#46, male)

This comment suggests that people do not always place their health as a first priority, especially when money is tight and they have a family to think about. Some 13% of our sample still had dependent children living at home with them.

Several participants described how they found "it very costly to pay for my medication that I will be taking for the rest of my life" (#42, male). This can be particularly problematic when patients are on several medications because they may have to choose between them. Other participants were upset that they were experiencing unnecessary side effects from having to go on the cheaper version of their medication. For example, one woman describes her situation.

> Well, you know, the biggest problem there is cost. The tablets that you are taking are the cheapest they can pay for. There was an article last week that I read about statins; especially synthastatin, which is the cheapest one, is actually causing deaths. And the statins that do work are about 6 times to 8 times dearer. So you won't get them. Originally I was on one statin and then they changed me over to synthastatin obviously because it was the cheaper option. (#14, male)

Although the actual cost of the medications are covered by the NHS, many people still have to pay the dispensing fee which can quickly add up. At least 36% of this sample did not qualify for an exemption from paying the dispensing fees. One man described how he requires 10 prescribed items per month (at £6.85 per item = £68.50) to manage his heart disease. He said that "it is extremely difficult to meet that cost out of my income. Other things have to be forfeited." Others who have even more chronic illnesses may have even more difficulties, especially if they cannot afford the lump sum for the "pre-payment certificate" (which helps to spread the cost).

A key message in most chronic disease management programs is to eat a healthy, well-balanced diet. What is often not recognized is that such foods are often expensive and not always within reach of those who are deprived. Several of the participants felt that eating low fat meats, fruits, and vegetables was too expensive for them. For instance, one man told us how he would "love to be able to buy low fat meat but I can't afford it" (#36, male). Another woman similarly claimed, "If you are on a low income with a little family you can relate to why we buy the cheaper foods" (#44, male). It is not easy to lead a healthy lifestyle on a small income. Participants often found it stressful that they were being told to eat healthier when they could not afford it.

> Now how many of you are told you've got to be on this diet? You can't have this, you can't have that and not one of us get any extra help because if you stick to that diet religiously, it cost's you a damn site more. (#27, male)

Some described how they would change their diet to include a lot more healthy foods if they had more money.

> I'd be at Morrison's fish counter every day if I could afford to buy a nice piece of cod, hake, haddock or salmon and alternatively lean steak, organic chicken and rack of lamb and lots of more exotic fruits and vegetables. If I had money my current food shopping list would change 100%. (#43, male)

Another man also said that he would "like to eat more fruit and vegetables but I'm on a tight budget and I consider that an extra" (#31, male). This was witnessed first-hand at the focus groups that were conducted where several people left the meetings actually filling their pockets with food. One man told me afterwards that it was the first time that he had ever tasted a kiwi while others said it has been ages since they had this selection of fruit. It was evident that many of these people were not able to afford a healthy well-balanced diet.

A key indictor of social class is employment status. Given the age of this sample and the extent of their heart problems, many of them had to retire early, which often had a profound impact on their self-esteem and mental well-being. One man describes how he felt when his doctor told him he could no longer work.

> You say to your doctors and your specialists: I feel great now can I go back to work and they turn around and say "no, not in the slightest chance." If you go back to work we'll

sign you off our book and have nothing more to do with you. It's bad news. You're a useless person. (#76, male)

Another man agreed and said, "you feel guilty about it. You can't support your family" (#42, male). Indeed, it may have been difficult for these people to stay motivated to manage their health when they were feeling upset about no longer being employed.

Another barrier related to their social class was that many of the patients in this sample relied on public transport either because they could no longer drive or because they did not own a car. One particular man who was no longer able to drive his car experienced a substantial blow to his confidence and sense of independence. He said, "the main thing is that they have told me that I am not to drive anymore" (#78, male). When this happens you not only have to deal with the practicalities of how you are going to get around but you also lose your sense of independence.

Public transportation is not always cheap either and several people complained about the rising fares and felt this was a barrier in getting around.

I noticed in the Advertiser today that the concessionary fares on the buses are going up to 70 p, a rise of 40%. It's not too bad for those who get free fares after 9.30 am and at weekends but what about a family with 3 kids at school? If my math is right they will now have to pay out at least £21 a week in bus fares. (#46, male)

Rising transportation fees could create problems for those who are on a small budget. Many of these participants encountered transportation problems while managing their heart problems. For example, many of the participants were either too old to drive or did not own a car. Thus, they had to rely on public transport which was not always affordable or accessible.

You see we've only got 1 bus an hour. We're very badly off the buses. So I couldn't have gone out this morning. For getting anywhere really. So I suppose that dominates my life more than anything. (#39, female)

I can't get out to the [cardiac] exercise classes because I can't drive and the classes aren't on an accessible bus route. (#20, female)

Women who lived on their own often did not want to venture too far from home.

I don't know how I'd get to cardiac rehab. I think you go into Eccles and then from Eccles you would get the 68, but that's far too far for me. (#84, female)

A lot of the participants would plan their activities around whether or not it was accessible by bus. "I was just thinking if I could get there with my bus pass" (#22, male).

Several people said how it was difficult getting out and about, especially to the doctors or to cardiac rehabilitation. Even when financial help is available to help offset the cost of transport to medical appointments there are still many difficulties encountered. One woman describes her difficulties with attending health appointments.

> I have gotten round the problems of attending hospital appointments by using G.M. Transport taxi vouchers. In theory I should be entitled to either book transport through my GP or claim back the cost of transport. The reality is that booked transport can add many hours on waiting time (almost 5 on the occasion I tried it) and the office for claiming back fares is often miles away from outpatients. At Hope Hospital it is part of the old building and at a recent appointment at St. Mary's it was over a mile away and of course you have to remember to keep all your receipts. Yesterday an appointment at Manchester Royal Infirmary cost me £26 return taxi fare. (#23, female)

The costs and hassles in simply getting to the hospital via public transport for routine appointments can add stress to patients and possibly hinder their motivation for actively managing their heart conditions. Indeed, some people told us how they were frustrated with trying to find parking near the hospital. Others talked about their concern with being sent to hospitals that were not near to where they lived, which added stress in figuring out how to get there. Thus, transportation problems seemed to be a main concern influencing people's ability to manage their CHD.

Age-Related Barriers

Most of the participants felt that managing their health was increasingly difficult to as they aged. For example, they felt that they did not have as much energy anymore to cope with everything.

> It feels like at 60, now I'm 65, feels like someone through this book at you and said, that's it; you've got to be ill now. (#34, male)

Many people described how they were quite frustrated with this. Some viewed their bodies more mechanically and said it was a matter of the "engine breaking down" while for others it was exhausting dealing with multiple chronic health problems.

> I think it's accepting that the engine is wearing down and you just can't run. It's hard because if you are bored, if you've got an active mind, you are still 18 aren't you? You want to do it and that's what gets you down. (#44, female)

> The things I could do 15–20 years ago I find difficult now. But I put this down to old age rather than my heart condition. (#54, male)

Indeed, some felt quite upset and depressed at times over their inability to do some of the things they used to do. The participants often found it difficult to accept that they were limited because of their health. One of the problems with aging is that their memory was not as good as it used to be. This can be particularly problematic when trying to remember when to take your medications.

> I mostly forget to take my medication in a morning because I must eat before I take them. I cannot eat first thing in a morning so I do everything else first and often forget, and it's not till the evening my body reminds me. (#42, male)

One man described how he tried to deal with this problem.

> I tried one of those marked daily trays to put your tablets in but I found it too fiddly. I sometimes forget but I don't think forgetting a dose now and then is that crucial accept for my warfarin to keep my blood levels right. There's times when my tablets have ran out and I couldn't get my prescription for a couple of days. (#43, male)

Such age-related problems can influence people's ability to manage health. Contending with all of these problems can leave patients feeling very exhausted with little energy to effectively manage their health.

> I do suffer with side effects of the disease, namely coughing, especially in bed, swollen ankles due to water retention, loss of appetite. I am never hungry and finally, tiredness. I can be active all day, but if I stop and sit down, I usually fall asleep. (#28, male)

Others encountered difficulties with their daily activities.

> I can't even lift myself out of the bath. My muscles have literally disappeared. They cause me a lot of knee problems because I've gone so thin here, the muscle is disappearing and I'm going weaker ... and I haven't slept properly for about 3 years. (#75, male)

Effectively managing your health may be difficult when your body is not able to function as it used to. Another man describes his frustration:

> What does cheese me off and sometimes gets me down is when I do things like, for example, when I chased my granddaughter down the garden path, picked her up and "monstered" her then had to use my GTN and sit down for 10 minutes to recover. Sometimes it's impossible to avoid difficult situations and who'd want to avoid one like that any way? It's worth an hour's angina to see her laugh like that. (#46, male)

This example suggests that it is often difficult to manage chronic illness when you want to keep living a "normal" life.

Several participants found it difficult to manage their health because they were contending with several chronic problems (mainly arthritis and diabetes). For example, it is difficult to exercise more often when you are in too much pain from the arthritis. One woman explains

> I know I'm carrying a lot of weight but that is due to painful knees. It is one vicious circle. Once you start not being able to exercise because of your mobility you start to put on the weight. The weight aggravates your arthritis and round and round you go. You try to keep as mobile as you can, but some days the pain that you have makes it difficult. (#44, female)

With this kind of pain experienced due to arthritis it is difficult to get the recommended level of exercise to maintain a healthy lifestyle. Many patients also found it incredibly frustrating when their doctors would tell them to simply get more exercise and lose weight. Yet, they could not easily do this because of the pain they were in, which often made all their health problems worse. Others were in a similar situation: "I could hardly walk. Walking up the stairs was like knives going into my knees. I was in agony" (#54, male). One man described how his inability to exercise was causing him to put on weight.

> I now have the knee syndrome which prevents long walks which for a long time levelled out my weight. I use to walk my dogs 5 to 10 miles a day without any effort in my 20s and 30s. (#43, male)

Over 40% of people with multiple chronic illnesses in this sample were told by their GP to get more exercise despite the limitations and pain they experienced. In sum, having a chronic condition is not always easy to contend with as you age because your body is wearing down, tiring easily and often encountering multiple health problems.

Barriers Stemming from Marital Status

Marital status often came up as a key theme that influenced people's self-management of their health. At this age many of the participants were having to look after their ill spouses or having to deal with them passing away. One woman describes her experience after her husband died.

> I was very happily married until 18 months ago when my husband died. I have been ill for 25 years not just with heart problems. I suffer with angina. I have had a mild heart attack and have ended up in intensive care. I am very, very lonely and I am very restricted because I can't drive. (#56, female)

For this woman, she did not realize how much she relied on her husband for support and found it difficult to manage everything on her own. Another woman describes how she felt after her husband passed away.

> When you are busy in your younger days, you do not make time for hobbies. You always say you haven't the time. Some people are fortunate enough to have a good

> marriage always doing things together, but when one or the other dies that is when the one left is at a loss as what to do with themselves. (#44, female)

Again, the theme of loneliness comes up which could have an influence on mental well-being and motivation to manage health. Women were not the only ones who experienced the passing of a loved one of this stage of life. Several men described how they were affected.

> It's a horrible time when a loved one dies and it affects you in many ways. My mum died 2 and a half years ago. She was 88 and had a peaceful death. My ex-wife died last year. We were again good friends. She had a long illness and a very difficult death. I was glad I was around to help my kids through it. They are all in their 30s but each took it very badly. (#46, male)

Another man describes his experience after his wife died.

> Two years ago, unfortunately I lost my wife after 43 years of marriage. The doctor says to me, you know, one thing you mustn't do, it mustn't get you stressed out. We have been down this road before we don't want to go down the road again. (#14, male)

Indeed, the death of a spouse can create a lot of distress and may worsen symptoms of those who already have heart problems. Although each person dealt with the death of their spouse in a different way it shaped the way that they thought about their illness and the priority it took in their life.

Some participants described how they did not actively manage their health because they were too busy looking after their spouse.

> I have a problem with my wife. She is disabled. She has COPD. It is a killer which is the gradual deterioration of your lungs. She's only got 35% of her lungs left. It's a terrible disease. There's nothing you can do about it actually. She's down to the point now that when we go shopping, every 10 yards she has to stop and catch her breath. It does cause a bit of a problem in that respect. (#87, male)

Somewhat surprising, the results from our questionnaire show that a significantly lower proportion of those who lived on their own were referred to cardiac rehabilitation (28.5%) compared to those who were married (65.6%) ($p < .05$). It is difficult to tell whether the inequality existed at the health provider level or whether single people were less likely to attend in the first place. Furthermore, a significantly higher proportion of those who were single visited the emergency department for their heart conditions (84.6%) compared to those who were married (3.3%) ($p < .001$). It could be that those who have the support and encouragement of a partner may be more inclined to visit their GP regularly and thus, not needing to go to emergency as often. Those who were married reported having significantly more social support compared to those who were single ($p < .01$). This support may prove to be quite beneficial for managing health because a partner can provide both practical and emotional support.

Gender-Related Barriers and Inequalities

The data show that several gender differences were present in terms of self-managing of CHD. Living on your own with fewer social supports may affect people's ability and motivation to manage their illness. In our sample, women were more likely to live on their own where only 28.6% of them were married compared to 70.8% of men. This is further exacerbated by women's significantly lower average household incomes (£7,800) compared to men (£13,000).

The symptoms of CHD are often different for women and most participants described how they were shocked by their diagnosis as they "thought it was a man's disease" (#16, female). In fact, a few of the women in the project were retired nurses who did not recognize the symptoms of their heart attack because they tend to be different for women.

> When I had my heart attack I didn't think for one minute it was a heart attack and as the day went on I didn't feel very well. I said to my husband I'd been sick, which I am never, ever sick and he said, oh that's a bit worrying so we went to the hospital and I'd had a heart attack. It never, ever occurred to me and I was a trained heart care nurse, which is a bit scary. (#23, female)

Some women said that they felt

> Just isolated, just left behind. Well, they say you get all these other symptoms and you don't know whether it's your heart or whether it's just getting old. (#35, female)

Indeed, many women claimed that they "definitely have different symptoms than men" (#82, female). This can have implications for diagnosis, treatment, and how the disease is managed.

Others highlighted the gender inequalities that they noticed in terms of the risk of heart disease being emphasized to their sons and not to their daughters.

> My 2 sons are on low doses of statins, not in response to any major problems but suggested by their respective doctors as precautionary because of family history. They didn't suggest anything similar to my daughters. (#46, male)

This is somewhat alarming that this kind of gender bias in treatment still occurs because it can delay diagnosis and treatment. Indeed, during the recruitment phase of the project some of the GPs who helped us to select our sample said that we need not bother to include women in our trial because heart disease is a man's problem!

The gendered division of labor can also influence self-management of health. One woman told us about the stress she encountered while looking after her husband.

> My husband said to me that I've spent so much of my life looking after him that it was now my turn. The only thing about all of this is that 2 months after he died I got all of this. Then I was annoyed. (#89, female)

It could be that this woman did not have much time to take care of her own health and so the stress and exhaustion of care giving built up over time. Some women described how they still had to keep up with the chores despite their illness.

> It's hard cooking dinner when you are not well. My partner cannot cook. All he can cook is sausage, eggs and chips. That's another worry is that he's not going to get out to eat when I'm in the hospital because he can't cook. So I always make sure there are meals in the freezer for him. (#56, female)

Such gendered roles can add stress for women because they may prioritize their family's needs over their own health. In the particular case of heart disease women may be at a disadvantage because their economic and social circumstances likely influence their ability to manage their health.

DISCUSSION

The purpose of this chapter was to explore the social barriers and inequalities that patients encounter while self-managing their heart condition. The focus was on an elderly sample from a deprived, inner city area of Greater Manchester, UK. This is salient because there has been a lack of attention paid to the role of social class, gender, and age on people's ability to self-manage their health. Most studies have tended to focus on middle-class samples while less is known about those who live in deprived urban areas. Further, past research has focused on inequalities in managing diabetes and arthritis while less attention has been paid to people managing heart disease.

These results suggest that these heart patients experienced many barriers and social inequalities that influenced their ability to manage their health. Social class, transportation problems, age, gender, and marital status were all key factors that influenced patient's ability to manage their heart problems. Since most of our sample was considered to be deprived they encountered many challenges with maintaining a healthy lifestyle, especially purchasing a well-balanced diet.

The findings in relation to affording prescriptions may seem somewhat surprising given the relatively generous nature of the NHS; however, there are people who do fall between the gaps. Although patients do not pay for the cost of their medications, like they do in America, most do have to pay the dispensing fee of £6.85 per item. Prescription charges were initially implemented to deter unnecessary prescribing and keep NHS costs down; however, many health groups now claim that prescription charges (dispensing fee) are having a negative effect on health, especially for those who are on low incomes (Fox, 2007; National Health Service (NHS), 2007). A report by the National Association of Citizens Advice Bureau (2001) claimed that nearly 750,000 prescriptions in England and Wales were not dispensed because people could not afford it. Research in the UK, Europe, and Canada consistently show that prescription charges result in patients not taking the medications they require, or even rationing their medication because of cost (NHS, 2007; Schafheutle, 2003). In the UK, some argue that patients can simply use a "pre-payment certificate" which spreads the cost of their prescriptions; yet many people were not able to benefit from this scheme because they could not afford the lump-sum payments (National Association of Citizen Advice Bureau, 2001). This is very concerning because lacking a prescription benefit is often linked with difficulty affording medications (Saver, Doescher, Jackson, & Fishman, 2004).

In 2001 in the UK, only about half of those who applied for the low income scheme (to help get their prescriptions paid for) received help (Sihota, 2003). Meanwhile, those who had incomes just above exemption levels reported how prescriptions costs "can quickly become unaffordable" (Sihota, 2003). This is especially problematic for disadvantaged groups because they are more likely to experience ill health. Although such problems are often more extreme in America (Blendon et al., 2002) there are many patients in the UK who are also struggling to pay for their prescriptions. Thus, prescription charges may end up compounding the cycle of health inequality for disadvantaged groups.

Others described how they often had to prioritize their family's needs over their own health when decisions had to be made about how to spend their small income. Indeed, worrying about the basic necessities of life may hinder people's ability to manage their health by adding stress, which may even worsen their heart symptoms. This is consistent with past research which shows that those who have higher incomes often engage in better self-care (Prus, 2007). Those who are from lower socio-economic backgrounds often lack the resources to properly self-manage their condition such as buying healthy foods and having reliable transport to get to medical appointments.

Many of the people in this study relied on public transportation and found it difficult to visit their physician and to attend cardiac rehabilitation exercise classes because they were often not readily accessible on a bus route and a taxi would be too costly for them. This can be problematic and lead to further health problems (Todd, Read, Lacey, & Abbott, 2001). This is consistent with past research showing that transportation problems often place people at a disadvantage in monitoring their health (Bayliss et al., 2003; Jerant et al., 2006). Research by the Social Exclusion Unit shows that people relying on public transport are restricted in taking up health promotion services (HM Treasury and Department of Health, 2002). For example, 27% of those in the UK who do not have a car have difficulty traveling to the hospital (Sihota, 2003). Thus, access to health services and reliable transport is not only a problem for people in rural areas but within inner cities as well.

As people age, they are likely to experience multiple chronic health problems, and changes in living conditions (especially marital status). Many people found it difficult to get more exercise to help keep their heart fit because they were contending with arthritis. This is consistent with past research showing that elderly persons often require more assistance to self-manage their conditions because they often contend with several conditions (Beckman et al., 2005; Elzen et al., 2007). Health care providers should keep in mind that it is not always easy for people to simply get more exercise when they are in a great deal of pain.

Marital status also played a significant part of their ability to manage their health as many of them were either caring for an ill spouse or had recently dealt with their death. Such a change in living conditions can influence practical every day activities like shopping and cooking and it may also influence how they prioritize their illness. Others (e.g., Christian et al., 2007; Soubhi et al., 2006) also found that those who live on their own may encounter more difficulties with their health.

Several inequalities were also experienced by gender, especially for women as they are more likely to live on their own and with a smaller income. Women tend to care for other family members and continue with the household chores despite their heart condition. Thus, their own health was often not as high of a priority for them. This is similar to Townsend, Wyke, & Hunt (2006)who found that patients often prioritize other social roles such as parenting or caring for a spouse over their own health.

What is evident from this research is that social inequalities often overlap and influence each other. This was particularly the case from this deprived, urban sample where having a low income seemed to worsen other social inequalities. Age, gender, social class, and marital status can influence life experiences, access to resources and thus, ability to manage health. People from deprived, inner city areas such as this sample, may lack resources and control over their life circumstances to be able to manage their health effectively. Their social position may leave them vulnerable to a negative cumulative effect and poorer access to resources to facilitate a healthy lifestyle (Prus, 2007).

In conclusion, several inequalities exist in self-managing heart disease. The process of self-management could be eased if the broader social and cultural context in which it takes place are addressed (Townsend et al., 2006). Addressing such inequalities is important to help improve patient's well-being and to reduce the burden on the health care system. Health care providers should also be cognizant of such social barriers that patients may face when engaging in self-care and give them the support and resources that they need to maintain their health.

ACKNOWLEDGMENTS

The funding for this project was provided by the Economic and Social Research Council within its "e-society" program and the HEFCE Social Research Infrastructure Fund. The author acknowledges the broader influence of Paul Bellaby, Simon Smith, and Frances Bell. I would also like to thank the project staff Safeena Aslam, George Gergianakis, and Peter Lok for all of their hard work. An earlier version of this chapter was presented at the *ESRC Symposium: Barriers and Inequalities in Self-Managing Chronic Illness*, Think Lab, Salford UK, May 11, 2007.

REFERENCES

Bayliss, E., Steiner, J., Fernald, D., Crane, L., & Main, D. (2003). Descriptions of barriers to self-care by persons with comorbid chronic diseases. *Annals of Family Medicine*, *1*(1), 15–21.

Beckman, A., Bernsten, C., Parker, M., Thorslund, M., & Fastbom, J. (2005). The difficulty of opening medicine containers in old age. *Pharmacy World and Science, 27*(5), 393–398.

Bell, E., & Orpin, P. (2006). Self management of chronic conditions: Implications for rural physicians of a demonstration project down under. *Canadian Journal of Rural Medicine, 11*(1), 33–40.

Bentley, J. (2003). Barriers to accessing health care: The perspective of elderly people within a village community. *International Journal of Nursing Studies, 40*(1), 9–21.

Blendon, R., Schoen, C., DesRoches, C., Osborn, R., Scoles, K., & Zapert, K. (2002). Inequities in health care: A five-country survey. *Health Affairs, 21*(5), 182–191.

British Heart Foundation. (2005). *Coronary heart disease statistics.* www.heartstats.org

Canadian Health Services Research Foundation. (2007). *Self-management education to optimize health and reduce hospital admissions for chronically ill patients.* Evidence Boost for Quality. CHSRF, June. http://www.chsrf.ca/mythbusters/pdf/boost10_e.pdf

Christian, A., Cheema, H., Smith, A., & Mosca, S. (2007). Predictors of quality of life among women with coronary heart disease. *Quality of Life Research, 16*(3), 363–373.

Curtis, J. (2003). *Social inequality in Canada.* Toronto: Pearson.

D'Arcy, C. (1998). Social distribution of health. In: Coburn, D'Arcy & Torrance (Eds), *Health and Canadian society: Sociological perspectives.* Toronto: University of Toronto Press.

Dannefer, D. (2003). Cumulative advantage/disadvantage and life curse: Cross-fertilizing age and social science theory. *Journal of Gerontology, 58,* S327–S337.

Elzen, H., Slaets, J., Snijders, T., & Steverink, N. (2007). Evaluation of the chronic disease self-management program among chronically ill older people in the Netherlands. *Social Science and Medicine, 64,* 1832–1841.

Fiscella, K., Franks, P., Gold, M., & Clancy, C. (2000). Inequality in quality: Addressing socioeconomic, racial and ethnic disparities in health care. *Journal of the American Medical Association, 283,* 2579–2584.

Fox, C. (2007). *Charges undermine free healthcare principle.* Scottish Socialist Party. http://www.scottishsocialistparty.org/scrap/scrap01.html

Green, J., & Thorogood, N. (2004). *Qualitative methods for health research.* London: Sage Publications.

Greene, J., & Yedidia, M. (2005). Provider behaviours contributing to patient self-management of chronic illness among underserved populations. *Journal of Health Care for the Poor and Underserved, 16,* 808–824.

Griffiths, C., Motlib, J., Azad, A., Ramsay, J., Eldridge, S., Feder, G., Khanam, R., Munni, R., Garrett, M., Turner, A., & Barlow, J. (2005). Randomised controlled trial of a lay-led self-management programme for Bangladeshi patients with chronic disease. *British Journal of General Practice, 55*(520), 831–837.

HM Treasury and Department of Health. (2002). *Tackling health inequalities: Cross-cutting review.*

Jerant, A., von Friederichs-Fitzwater, M., & Moore, M. (2006). Patients perceived barriers to active self-management of chronic conditions. *Patient Education and Counselling, 57,* 300–307.

King, K., Thomlinson, E., Sanguins, J., & LeBlanc, P. (2006). Men and women managing coronary artery disease risk: Urban–rural contrasts. *Social Science and Medicine, 62,* 1091–1102.

Lindsay, S. (2007). Decision-making and expert patients. Expert commentary. In: P. Tolana (Ed.), *Decision making in medicine and health care.* New York: Nova Science Publishers.

Lindsay, S., Bellaby, P., Smith, S., & Baker, R. (2008). Enabling healthy choices: Is ICT the highway to health improvement? *Health: An interdisciplinary journal in the study of health and illness, 12*(3), 313–331.

Lindsay, S., Smith, S., Bell, F., & Bellaby, P. (2007). Tackling the digital divide: Exploring the impact of ICT on managing heart conditions. *Journal of Information, Communication and Society, 10*(1), 95–114.

Ljung, R., Peterson, S., Hallqvist, J., Heimerson, I., & Diderichsen, F. (2005). Socioeconomic differences in the burden of disease in Sweden. *Bulletin of the World Health Organization, 83*(2), 92–99.

McKinlay, J. (1996). Some contributions from the social system to gender inequalities in heart disease. *Journal of Health and Social Behavior, 37*(1), 1–26.

Nagelkerk, J., Reick, K., & Meengs, L. (2006). Perceived barriers and effective strategies to diabetes self-management. *Journal of Advanced Nursing, 54*(2), 151–158.

National Association of Citizens Advice Bureau. (2001). *Unhealthy charges: CAB evidence on the impact of health charges.*

National Health Service (NHS). (2007). *NHS prescription charges.* http://www.politics.co.uk/issue-briefs/health/nhs/nhs-prescription-services/nhs-prescription-charges-$366605.htm

Nolte, S., Elsworth, G., Sinclair, A., Osborne, J., & Richard, H. (2007). The extent and breadth of benefits from participating in chronic disease self-management courses: A national patient-reported outcomes survey. *Patient Education and Counselling, 65*(3), 351–360.

Peterson, S., Peto, V., & Rayner, M. (2004). *Coronary heart disease statistics.* University of Oxford: British Heart Foundation Health Promotion Research Group.

Pincus, T., Esther, R., DeWalt, D., & Callahan, L. (1998). Social conditions and self-management are more powerful determinants of health than access to care. *Annals of Internal Medicine, 129*, 406–411.

Prashar, A. (2000). *Coronary heart disease in the North West.* Public Health Information Report: North West Public Health Observatory.

Prus, S. (2007). Age, SES and health: A population level analysis of health inequalities over the lifecourse. *Sociology of Health and Illness, 29*(2), 275–296.

Richards, L. (1999). *Using NVIVO in qualitative research.* London: Sage Publications.

Richards, H., McConnachie, A., Morrison, C., Murray, K., & Watt, G. (2000). Social and gender variation in the prevalence, presentation and general practitioner provisional diagnosis of chest pain. *Journal of Epidemiology and Community Health, 54*, 714–718.

Salford City Council. (2005). *Strategic planning background.* http://www.salford.gov.uk/living/planning/udp/udpcurrent/udp-background.htm

Salford Primary Care Trust (PCT). (2005). *Improving the health of Salford.* Salford NHS PCT. http://www.salford-pct.nhs.uk/foi/our_services.asp?id = 6

Saver, B., Doescher, M., Jackson, J., & Fishman, P. (2004). Seniors with chronic health conditions and prescription drugs. *Value in Health, 7*(2), 133–143.

Schafheutle, E. (2003). Do high prescription charges undermine compliance? *The Pharmaceutical Journal, 270.*

Schofield, T. (2007). Health inequity and its social determinants: A sociological commentary. *Health Sociology Review, 16*(2), 105–114.

Sihota, S. (2003). *Creeping charges: NHS prescription, dental and optical charges – an urgent case for treatment.* National Consumer Council.

Singh-Manoux, A., Chandola, F., & Marmot, M. (2004). Socioeconomic trajectories across the life course and health outcomes in midlife: Evidence for the accumulation hypothesis? *International Journal of Epidemiology, 33,* 1072–1079.

Soubhi, H., Fortin, M., & Hudon, C. (2006). Perceived conflict in the couple and chronic illness management: Preliminary analyses from the Quebec Health Survey. *BMC Family Practice, 7,* 59.

Taylor, D., & Bury, M. (2007). Chronic illness, expert patients and care transition. *Sociology of Health and Illness, 29,* 27–45.

Todd, A., Read, C., Lacey, A., & Abbott, J. (2001). Barriers to uptake of services for coronary heart disease. *British Medical Journal, 323,* 1–5.

Townsend, P., & Davidson, N. (Eds). (1982). *Inequalities in health: The black report and the health divide.* Harmondsworth: Pelican.

Townsend, A., Wyke, S., & Hunt, K. (2006). Self-managing and managing the self: Practical and moral dilemmas in accounts of living with chronic illness. *Chronic Illness, 2,* 185–194.

Wilson, P., Kendall, S., & Brooks, F. (2007). The expert patients programme: A paradox of patient empowerment and medical dominance. *Health & Social Care in the Community* (in press).

Winters, C., Cudney, S., Sullivan, T., & Thuesen, A. (2006). The rural context and women's self-management of chronic health conditions. *Chronic Illness, 2*(4), 273–289.

FUNCTIONAL ABILITY AND DISABILITY AMONG OLDER ADULTS WITH ARTHRITIS: THE IMPACT OF AGE, DURATION OF ARTHRITIS, AND SEVERITY OF ARTHRITIS

Leah Rohlfsen and Jennie Jacobs Kronenfeld

ABSTRACT

Arthritis is the most prevalent chronic condition in persons ages 65 and older and is projected to increase substantially as the population ages. The purpose of this research is to assess if age, duration of arthritis, and severity of arthritis exert independent effects on various aspects of the disability process: functional limitations, activities of daily living (ADL) limitations, and instrumental activities of daily living (IADL) limitations. Type of arthritis, socio-demographic factors, behavioral factors, and additional health statuses are also examined. Using longitudinal data from the Health and Retirement study, results show age and severity of arthritis are related to the number of functional limitations one has and to

Care for Major Health Problems and Population Health Concerns:
Impacts on Patients, Providers and Policy
Research in the Sociology of Health Care, Volume 26, 41–64
Copyright © 2008 by Emerald Group Publishing Limited
All rights of reproduction in any form reserved
ISSN: 0275-4959/doi:10.1016/S0275-4959(08)26003-5

the odds of having ADL and IADL limitations. Duration of arthritis is positively related to functional limitations and to the odds of reporting ADL limitations. Duration of arthritis is not significantly related to IADL limitations, which are strongly linked to performing social roles and have less to do with physical functioning compared to ADL tasks and functional tasks. There is no difference between those with established arthritis compared to those who have had it for a shorter time period, suggesting those with arthritis adapt to social tasks better than physical tasks. The resources used to cope with IADL limitations may be more effective over time compared to those used to cope with functional limitations and ADL disability. Understanding the context of functional limitations and disability among those with arthritis may lead to improved support and care for those living with arthritis.

INTRODUCTION

Arthritis is the most prevalent chronic condition in persons ages 65 and older (Dunlop, Manheim, Song, & Chang, 2001; Dunlop, Manheim, Yelin, Song, & Chang, 2003b). In fact, the prevalence of self-reported, doctor-diagnosed arthritis is projected to increase from 47.8 million in 2005 to nearly 67 million by 2030 in the Unites States (Hootman & Helmick, 2006). Arthritis and other chronic conditions are long-term diseases and as the population ages, more people will have to live with arthritis for a longer period of time (Leveille, Wee, & Iezzoni, 2005). Furthermore, it is a leading cause of functional activity limitations among older adults and by 2030, 25 million are projected to report arthritis-attributable activity limitations (Hootman & Helmick, 2006).

According to Covinsky (2006), arthritis is often viewed as a benign condition because it is so ubiquitous among older adults and is rarely associated with mortality. Actually, arthritis can lead to physical and mental dysfunction, visits to health care workers, therapeutic regimes and surgical procedures, dependency on equipment or other people, hospital and nursing home stays, sadness and fear, and death (Verbrugge & Juarez, 2001; Verbrugge & Patrick, 1995). Research has shown that people with arthritis experience more depressive symptoms, less self-esteem, and a lower sense of control (Penninx et al., 1996). Arthritis can cause difficulty in performing roles and other valued activities. Evers, Kraaimaat, Geenen, Jacobs, and Bijlsma (2003) found that 75% of those with arthritis suffer from limitations affecting their leisure time and social activities. In addition, those with arthritis are substantial users of health care services (Dunlop, Manheim, Song, & Chang, 2003a; Dunlop et al., 2003b). Arthritis is responsible for 750,000 hospitalizations and 36 million outpatient visits every year (U.S. Department of Health and Human Services, 2005), and for major health care expenditures (Dunlop et al., 2003b; Vradenburg, Simoes, Jackson-Thompson, & Murayi, 2002). In 1997, the total cost of arthritis and other rheumatic conditions in the United States was $116.3 billion, with $51.1 billion in direct costs and $65.2 billion in indirect costs such as productivity and time loss (Centers for Disease Control and Prevention, 2003).

Medical and personal regimes can sometimes control, but rarely cure chronic diseases, such as arthritis. Although arthritis will essentially be a permanent feature in the lives of those who are diagnosed with it, certain socio-demographic characteristics, behaviors, and disease factors can make a difference in how arthritis impacts their lives. The focus of this research is to provide a comprehensive analysis of how different disease characteristics of arthritis affect various parts of the disability process. Research shows that age, duration of arthritis, and severity of arthritis are associated with physical functioning (Barlow, Cullen, & Rowe, 1999; Curtis, Groarke, Coughlan, & Gsel, 2004; Dunlop et al., 2003a; Fonseca, Canhao, Teixeira da Costa, da Silva, & Queiroz, 2002; Leigh, Fries, & Parikh, 1992; Long & Pavalko, 2004; Sheehan, DuBrava, Fifield, Reisine, & DeChello, 2004; Wray & Blaum, 2001). However, these studies examine age, duration, or severity independently and do not consider all three simultaneously. This research assesses if age, duration of arthritis, and severity of arthritis exert independent effects on physical functioning. Type of arthritis is also examined to see how various types of arthritis are related to physical functioning. In addition to the various disease characteristics, socio-demographic factors, behaviors, and additional health status characteristics are included in order to better understand how these factors impact physical functioning among those with arthritis.

Not only does this research focus on several aspects of arthritis, it considers various outcomes that are part of the disability process: functional limitations, activities of daily living (ADL) limitations, and instrumental activities of daily living (IADL) limitations. Most research has focused on the impact of rheumatoid arthritis on disability using the Health Assessment Questionnaire (HAQ) (Leigh & Fries, 1993; Leigh et al., 1992; Serbo & Jajic, 1991; Sheehan et al., 2004; Wolfe, 2000) . While useful, examining the impact of arthritis on different parts of the disability process can provide a more thorough understanding of how arthritis affects the lives of those with arthritis. Therefore, the purpose of this research is to examine the impact of age, duration, severity, and type of arthritis on functional limitations, ADL limitations, and IADL limitations using longitudinal data from the Heath and Retirement Study (HRS).

BACKGROUND

Past social science literature has primarily focused on the impact of arthritis on health care utilization and the economic costs of arthritis (Dunlop et al., 2003a, 2003b; Verbrugge & Patrick, 1995; Vradenburg et al., 2002). Although some research shows that those individuals with arthritis are likely to receive insufficient treatment and care (Leveille et al., 2005; Verbrugge & Patrick, 1995; Vradenburg et al., 2002), other research shows that those with arthritis are substantial users of health care services (Dunlop et al., 2003a, 2003b). Regardless of the utilization patterns of those with arthritis, the economic impact of arthritis is substantial and rising.

The association between arthritis and disability has been well documented (Dunlop et al., 2001; Hommel, Wagner, Chaney, White, & Mullins, 2004; Kosorok, Omenn, Diehr, Koepsell, & Patrick, 1992; Verbrugge, 1992; Verbrugge & Patrick, 1995; Vradenburg et al., 2002). Elderly people with arthritis are much more likely to have limitations in mobility and ADLs compared to elderly without arthritis (Dunlop et al., 2001; Verbrugge & Juarez, 2001; Verbrugge & Patrick, 1995). A comprehensive review of studies by Dunlop et al. (2003b) indicates that more than one-fifth of people with arthritis are unable to perform major activities of daily life. These include disabilities in the areas of work, mobility, activities, and ADLs. ADL limitations specifically were reported by one-third to half of people over 70 years of age with arthritis. For middle and late life, arthritis ranks first for limitations among both women and men (Verbrugge & Patrick, 1995). Limitations in performing basic functional tasks are particularly serious, because these limitations threaten the ability of adults to live independently.

An association between the severity of arthritis and functional limitations has been documented (Curtis et al., 2004; Dunlop et al., 2003a; Vradenburg et al., 2002). As severity of arthritis increases, physical functioning declines. However, it may not only be severity that impacts functional activity (Barlow et al., 1999; Treharne, Kitas, Lyons, & Booth, 2005). Duration may affect physical functioning. One set of beliefs posits that levels of functional ability and activity decrease as one lives with the chronic disease because of fear-avoidance (Evers et al., 2003) and losses in physical functioning as the illness progresses (Zimmer, Hickey, & Searle, 1997). Research confirms a positive relationship between duration and physical disability among those with rheumatoid arthritis (Barlow et al., 1999; Fonseca et al., 2002; Leigh et al., 1992; Sheehan et al., 2004). Similarly, Serbo and Jajic (1991) found that patients with long-term duration considered their functional abilities to be worse compared to those with short-term duration.

The other set of beliefs concerns the degree to which those with arthritis have adapted to their condition (Barlow et al., 1999). Individuals can vary greatly in their adaptation to disease and this is not always well explained by the severity of the disease (Curtis, Groarke, Coughlan, & Gsel, 2005). Duration of disease may affect how one learns to live and function with the disease, therefore increasing one's ability to perform activities. Those with arthritis obtain more useful knowledge and make more informed decisions concerning treatment and self-care activities. These adjustments may counteract physical loss, resulting in a positive relationship between duration of disease and physical functioning. Other research suggests that there is no relationship between duration and arthritis. In the first year of disease, levels of functioning and pain are comparable to that of patients with longstanding rheumatoid arthritis (Evers, Kraaimaat, Geenen, & Bijlsma, 1998; Meenan, Kazis, Anthony, & Wallin, 1991), suggesting that there are no differences in functioning by duration of disease among those with rheumatoid arthritis.

There is the possibility that duration may not be independently related to physical functioning once age and severity are taken into consideration. The studies that have considered how duration of arthritis is related to physical functioning do not include a measure of severity, or do not include a wide variety of potential confounding variables which may explain the relationship between duration and physical functioning (Barlow et al., 1999; Fonseca et al., 2002; Leigh et al., 1992; Serbo & Jajic, 1991; Sheehan et al., 2004).

Age has been shown to be a strong predictor of functional limitations and disability (Long & Pavalko, 2004; Wray & Blaum, 2001). Still, research shows that the functional decline commonly associated with age is not a direct consequence of age per se, but results from certain conditions such as arthritis, which are strongly associated with age (Kosorok et al., 1992). The impact of arthritis on activity limitations and the potential to cause disability rises with age (Gill, Robison, & Tinetti, 1998; Verbrugge & Patrick, 1995). Because of the strong correlation between age and duration of arthritis, it is important to determine if there are independent effects of duration of arthritis on physical functioning that are not a result of age, and vice versa. Sheehan et al. (2004) found that duration of illness is a better predictor of functional limitations than age, which runs counter to a finding by Wolfe (2000), who concluded that duration of arthritis was only weakly related to functional limitations. Fonseca et al. (2002) found that both disease duration and age are major factors predicting functional status of patients with rheumatoid arthritis, but did not examine severity of arthritis.

The majority of research on the impact of arthritis on physical functioning has focused on physician diagnosed rheumatoid arthritis (Barlow et al., 1999; Curtis et al., 2004, 2005; Evers et al., 1998, 2003; Fonseca et al., 2002; Hommel et al., 2004; Leigh & Fries, 1993; Leigh et al., 1992; Meenan et al., 1991; Serbo & Jajic, 1991; Sheehan et al., 2004; Treharne, Lyons, Booth, Mason, & Kitas, 2004; Treharne et al., 2005; Wolfe, 2000). Although osteoarthritis is the most common form of arthritis in older adults, research on rheumatoid arthritis is more extensive compared to osteoarthritis (Covinsky, 2006). Covinsky, Lindquist, Dunlop, Gill, and Yelin (2008) note that other types of conditions may be highly variable in their effect on functional limitations and disability. For example, Yelin, Lubeck, Holman, and Epstein (1987) studied the activity levels among those with rheumatoid arthritis and osteoarthritis, and concluded that those with rheumatoid arthritis experienced more activity losses than those with osteoarthritis. It is important to differentiate types of arthritis because they exhibit different patterns and may lead to differences on the outcomes (Yelin, 1992).

Similarly, most of the studies use clinical or small non-representative samples (Barlow et al., 1999; Fonseca et al., 2002; Leigh & Fries, 1993; Leigh et al., 1992; Serbo & Jajic, 1991; Sheehan et al., 2004; Treharne et al., 2004, 2005; Wolfe, 2000). Research has shown that reliance on physician diagnosis of arthritis underestimates the population prevalence of arthritis (Vradenburg et al., 2002). Although self-reports lack diagnostic accuracy, they are relevant because many persons with arthritis do not see a health care provider for their symptoms and it is appropriate to rely on self-reported data to measure the full burden of the disease (Dunlop et al., 2003b, 2001; Leveille et al., 2005). This study will utilize self-reported, non-physician diagnosed arthritis or rheumatism, as well as self-reported physician diagnosed arthritis or rheumatism. Furthermore, the analysis is based on a nationally representative sample of non-institutionalized older adults which allows us to use the results of this study to make generalizations about how arthritis affects physical functioning among non-institutionalized older adults in the United States.

The Disability Process

According to Nagi (1976), active pathology or disease leads to physiological, mental, or emotional impairment. Impairment in turn leads to functional limitations, which eventually result in disability. Functional limitations indicate difficulties with mobility, strength (large muscle functioning), gross motor skills, and fine motor skills (Fonda & Herzog, 2004) and link the breakdown of body function to disability (Johnson & Wolinsky, 1993, 1994; Verbrugge & Jette, 1994). It is important to note that not all impairments result in functional limitations, and not all functional limitations result in disability.

The measurement of functional limitations varies widely.[1] Some measure functional limitations based on Rosow and Breslau's (1966) index of three tasks: doing heavy work around the house, walking a half a mile, and going up and down stairs. However, measurement of functional limitations based on Nagi's (1976) index of functional limitations has become more common. His index assessed respondent's ability to perform seven physical activities and respond to eight emotional factors. Researchers have more recently divided the physical functional limitations into upper body components and lower body components (Clark, Stump, & Wolinsky, 1997; Johnson & Wolinsky, 1993, 1994). However, there are discrepancies as to which factors indicate which component. Long and Pavalko (2004) found the distinction between lower body and upper body limitations unnecessary. There continues to be variation in the indicators that are used to measure disability and functional limitations (Parker & Thorslund, 2007). This variation surrounds which and how many activities should be included as indicators, as well as the wording of the items which assess functional health status.

Disability is often assessed with scales indicating ability to perform ADL and IADL. These scales assess the ability to perform a series of tasks that are essential to independent living. ADLs evaluate self-care tasks such as bathing, eating, and dressing, while IADLs assess more complex social behavior such as meal preparation and shopping. Generally, elderly individuals report difficulty with IADL tasks, such as doing housework or using transportation, before they report difficulty with ADL tasks (Gill, Robison, & Tinetti, 1998). Utilizing ADL and IADL scales can be problematic because the level of impairment measured is quite severe (Bruce, 2001; Clark et al., 1997; Verbrugge & Jette, 1994) and it has been argued that ADLs and IADLs offer a narrow view of physical limitations (Katz, 1995).

Some researchers combine ADL, IADL, and functional limitations items into a single scale to indicate disability or functional health (Kaplan, Strawbridge, Camacho, & Cohen, 1993). Several studies among adults with rheumatoid arthritis measure physical function with the HAQ, which measures eight general categories of physical performance: dressing, grooming, arising, eating, walking, hygiene, reaching, gripping, and outside activities (Leigh & Fries, 1993; Leigh et al., 1992; Serbo & Jajic, 1991; Sheehan et al., 2004; Wolfe, 2000). Treharne and colleagues (2004) note that although the HAQ is a suitable measure of physical health limitations caused by rheumatoid arthritis, other measures of disability may highlight key aspects of disability other than those that are captured by the HAQ. Functional limitations indicate basic physical ability that may lead to more serious disability. ADL limitations indicate severe physical disability in tasks that prevent independent functioning, while IADLs indicate severe disability with social tasks.

Focusing on several outcomes related to the disability process allows for a more thorough understanding of the impact of arthritis on physical functioning. Furthermore, assessing the independent effects of age, duration, severity, and type of arthritis will allow for a more thorough understanding of how each of these factors influences physical functioning among those with arthritis. This research will examine if having lived with arthritis for a more established length of time (more than 8 years) compared to having lived with arthritis for a shorter period of time (less than 8 years) is significantly related to functional ability and disability. In sum, this analysis will examine the impact of age, duration of arthritis, severity of arthritis, and type of arthritis on functional limitations, ADL limitations, and IADL limitations using data from a longitudinal panel study of older adults.

DATA AND METHODOLOGY

The data used in this analysis come from the HRS. The HRS is a US nationally representative panel study of health, retirement, and aging sponsored by the National Institute on Aging and coordinated by the Institute for Survey Research at the University of Michigan. The original wave of the HRS data was collected in 1992 and sampled 12,652 people in 7,608 households born from 1931 to 1941 and their spouses. In 1998, the HRS data was merged with the Study of Assets and Health Dynamics Among the Oldest Old (AHEAD), which was first collected in 1993 and sampled 8,222 respondents born in 1923 or earlier and their spouses. Two new subsamples were also added in 1998. The first included 2,320 respondents born from 1924 to 1930, and the second included 2,529 respondents born from 1942 to 1947. In 2004, a subsample of 3,340 adults born between 1948 and 1953 was added, so that the current HRS is a panel study of individuals older than 50 years in 2004.

Individuals were selected from a sample of housing units generated using a multi-stage, clustered area probability sample. Face-to-face, in-home interviews were conducted at baseline and follow-up telephone interviews occur every second year, with proxy interviews after death. The HRS includes an over-sampling of Hispanics, Blacks, and Florida residents. Weight, cluster, and stratification variables are used to correct for the complex sampling design using Stata Version 9.2 (Stata Corp, 2005). The subpopulation command in Stata is used to limit the analysis to all those who reported having arthritis in the 1998, 2000, 2002, or 2004 waves. A respondent was considered to have arthritis if they answered yes to a question that asked if the respondent has arthritis or a doctor has told them that they have arthritis or rheumatism. This resulted in a subsample of 11,316 respondents. By looking at only those with arthritis, comparisons can be made regarding how duration, severity, and type of arthritis impact function and disability for those with arthritis.

The dependent variables, which will be explained in detail below, are functional limitations, ADL limitations, and IADL limitations and are taken from the 2004 wave. The key independent variables include age, severity of arthritis, duration of arthritis, and type of arthritis. Severity of arthritis is measured in 2002 to ensure proper causal ordering. Duration of arthritis is measured using merged data from the 1998, 2000, 2002, and 2004 waves. Type of arthritis is measured in 2004 because information regarding specific type of arthritis was not available for all respondents in prior waves. All other independent variables are taken from the 2002 wave.

Dependent Variables

The activities that compose the functional limitations scale include walking several blocks, walking one block, sitting for about 2 hours, getting up from a chair after sitting for long periods, climbing several flights of stairs without resting, climbing one flight of stairs without resting, lifting or carrying weights over 10 lbs, stooping, kneeling, or crouching, reaching arms above shoulder level, pushing or pulling large objects, and picking up a dime from the table. Respondents were asked if they had difficulty with each task.

Possible responses were "yes," "no," "can't do," and "don't do." Respondents who answered "can't do" are coded "yes" and those who answered "don't do" are coded as missing. All activities are dichotomous with zero equal to no limitation in the task and one equal to limitation in the task. They are combined into an additive scale with values ranging from zero to eleven.[2] The reliability for the functional limitations scale has been assessed with Chronbach's alpha and is .89 for the 2004 scale (Fonda & Herzog, 2004).

The ADL limitations scale is composed of the following tasks: dressing, walking, bathing, eating, getting in or out of bed, and using the toilet. Tasks indicating IADLs include the following: preparing meals, grocery shopping, making phone calls, taking medication, and managing money. Similar to the functional limitations scale described above, respondents were asked if they had difficulty with each task and possible responses were "yes," "no," "can't do," and "don't do." Those who answered "can't do" are coded "yes" and those who answered "don't do" are coded as missing. As a result, all tasks were dichotomous with zero equal to no limitation in the task and one equal to limitation in the task. All of the tasks are combined into an additive scale, with possible scores for the ADL outcome ranging from zero to six and possible scores for the IADL outcome ranging from zero to five. Because very few respondents have many ADL and IADL limitations, the measures were recoded into binary variables so that zero indicates no ADL or IADL limitations and one indicates limitation. The reliability for the ADL and IADL scales have been assessed with Chronbach's alpha and are .84 and .85 in 2000, respectively (Fonda & Herzog, 2004).

Independent Variables

Age is a continuous variable. Severity of arthritis comes from the 2002 wave and is composed of the following four indicators: if the respondent was seen by a doctor specifically for his/her arthritis, if the respondent has stiffness, pain, or swelling of the joints due to arthritis, if the respondent takes any medications or treatments for their arthritis, and if the respondent has had surgery or joint replacement because of arthritis. Scores range from zero for not severe to four for very severe.

Data from the 1998, 2000, 2002, and 2004 waves were merged to indicate how long a respondent has reported having arthritis. The information comes from the question which indicates if a respondent has arthritis or has had a doctor told them that they have arthritis or rheumatism. If a respondent reported they had arthritis in 1998, 2000, 2002, and 2004 they are coded as a one, indicating they have established duration. If a respondent indicates they reported arthritis for fewer than four consecutive waves, they are coded as a zero to indicate they have shorter duration. Treharne et al. (2005) define established duration as having lived with rheumatoid arthritis for at least 7 years. Those who reported irregular patterns of arthritis, for example, reported arthritis in 2000 and 2004 but not in 2002 are not included in the measure so that the measure of arthritis indicates consecutive years the respondent reported arthritis. Similarly, those for whom information was missing on this variable are not included in the measure either.

In 2004, respondents were asked about having the following four possible types of arthritis: osteoarthritis, rheumatoid arthritis, gout or lupus, and arthritis due to an injury. Because respondents could report having two types of arthritis, it is necessary to recode the types of arthritis so respondents are only in one category. These recoded categories are as follows: (1) osteoarthritis, which includes those that have osteoarthritis and arthritis due to an injury and those with osteoarthritis and gout or lupus (reference group), (2) rheumatoid arthritis, which includes those with rheumatoid arthritis and osteoarthritis, those with rheumatoid arthritis and arthritis due to an injury, and those with rheumatoid arthritis and gout or lupus, (3) gout or lupus, which includes those with gout or lupus and arthritis due to an injury, and (4) arthritis due to an injury.

Additional independent variables include gender, racial and ethnic background, marital status, education, household income, net wealth, presence of health insurance, morbidity, self-rated sight, self-rated hearing, participation in physical activity, BMI (body mass index), and smoking status.

Gender is coded so zero indicates males and one indicates female. Race and ethnicity is a dichotomous variable with non-Hispanic white coded as zero and non-Hispanic black, Hispanic, and non-Hispanic other coded as one. Marital status is coded so that zero indicates separated, divorced, widowed, and never married and one indicates married.

Education is coded as a continuous variable indicating number of years of school completed. Household income is total household income during the last calendar year and is logged in order to correct for the skewed distribution. Net wealth is net household assets minus debt and is also logged. Household wealth is transformed by taking the absolute value of the negative values and obtaining the natural log of those values. These values are then reassigned as negative values and combined with the natural log of the positive values to produce both negative and positive natural logged values. Presence of health insurance is a dichotomous variables indicating if the respondent is covered by health insurance from his or her current or previous employer, his or her spouse's employer, by any government health insurance program, or any other health insurance.

Morbidity indicates the number of chronic health conditions ever diagnosed. The respondents were asked whether or not a doctor has ever told them they had the following conditions: high blood pressure or hypertension, diabetes or high blood sugar, cancer or a malignant tumor of any kind except skin cancer, chronic lung disease except asthma such as chronic bronchitis or emphysema, heart attack, coronary heart disease, angina, congestive heart failure, or other heart problems, stroke or transient ischemic attack, arthritis or rheumatism, and emotional, nervous, or psychiatric problems. The number of conditions one has been diagnosed with is summed. Self-rated sight and self-rated hearing come from questions in which respondents were asked to rate their hearing and their eyesight. Seeing impairment is coded from one to six, with one indicating the respondent is legally blind, two indicating poor eyesight and six indicating excellent eyesight. Hearing impairment is coded from one to five, with one indicating poor hearing ability and five indicating excellent hearing ability.

Physical activity is assessed by asking if the respondent participates in vigorous activity 3 or more times per week. Vigorous activity includes sports, heavy housework, or a job that involves physical labor. BMI is calculated by dividing weight by the square of height (weight/height^2). BMI is coded as four dummies indicating if a respondent is normal weight (BMI of 18.5–24.4, reference group), underweight (BMI of less than 18.5), overweight (BMI of 24.5–29.4), or obese (BMI above 29.4). Smoking behavior is assessed with two questions. The first assesses if the respondent ever smoked cigarettes and the second assesses if the respondent currently smokes cigarettes. Smoking behavior is coded into the following categories: never smoked (reference group), former smoker, and current smoker.

Descriptive statistics for those that have arthritis are presented in Table 1. The mean age is approximately 68 years old in 2002. There are more females compared to males (60.5%) and the majority of the sample is non-Hispanic white (81.9%). Most of the respondents are currently married (62.3%) rather than divorced, separated, widowed, or never married. The average number of years of schooling completed is 12.34 and almost all report having some form of health insurance (96%). On average, respondents have 1.48 chronic conditions and rate their eyesight and hearing as good. More than one-third participate in physical activity at least 3 times per week. A large percentage are overweight (37.6%) or obese (33.1%), while 27.6%

Table 1. Weighted Descriptive Statistics for those with Arthritis ($N = 11,316$).

	%	Mean	Std. Dev
Dependent Variables			
Functional Limitations		3.82	3.08
ADL Limitations	22.3		
IADL Limitations	21.4		
Independent Variables			
Age (uncentered)		67.78	10.65
Established Duration	79.1		
Severity of Arthritis		1.72	1.02
Type of Arthritis			
Osteoarthritis	60.1		
Rheumatoid	24.9		
Gout/Lupus	2.8		
Arthritis due to an Injury	12.3		
Gender (female)	60.5		
Race/Ethnicity (non-Hispanic whites)	81.9		
Marital Status (married)	62.3		
Education		12.34	3.09
Household Income (logged)		10.30	1.55
Net Wealth (logged)		11.02	4.02
Insurance	95.5		
# of Chronic Conditions		1.48	1.22
Self-Rated Sight		4.16	1.00
Self-Rated Hearing		3.33	1.08
Participation in Physical Activity	39.7		
BMI			
Underweight	1.7		
Normal weight	27.6		
Overweight	37.6		
Obese	33.1		
Smoking Status			
Current Smoker	14.1		
Former Smoker	45.1		
Never Smoked	40.9		

are normal weight and very few are underweight (1.7%). A larger percentage of respondents are former smokers (45.1%) and non-smokers (40.9%) compared to the percent that currently smoke (14.1%).

The majority of respondents report having arthritis for at least eight consecutive years (79.1%). On average, respondents report a severity level of 1.72. Of the possible types of arthritis, 60.1% have osteoarthritis, 24.9% have rheumatoid arthritis, 2.8% have gout or lupus, and 12.3% have arthritis due to an injury. The mean number of functional limitations is 3.82, while 22.3% report ADL limitations and 21.4% report IADL limitations.

RESULTS

To assess the impact of age, duration, severity, and type of arthritis on functional limitations, ordinary least squares regression is performed, while logistic regression is used to assess the impact on ADLs and IADLs.[3] Results of the analysis examining the effect of age, duration, severity, and type of arthritis on functional limitations are presented in Table 2.

There is a positive relationship between age and functional limitations, so for every year increase in age, older adults with arthritis have .037 more functional limitations even when controlling for differences in duration. In addition, duration of arthritis is positively related to functional limitations, so those with more established arthritis have .759 more functional limitations compared to those who have had arthritis for a shorter duration. These results provide evidence of independent effects of age and duration on functional limitations. Severity of arthritis is also positively related to functional limitations, so that for each unit increase in severity of arthritis, the number of functional limitations one has increases by .647. Of the various types of arthritis examined, those with gout or lupus have .752 fewer functional limitations than those with osteoarthritis.

Results from the logistic regression analysis examining the effects of age, duration, severity, and type of arthritis on ADL and IADL limitations are presented in Table 3. Both age and duration have significant and independent effects on ADL limitations. For every year increase in age, the odds of reporting ADL limitations increase by 2.5%. Furthermore, those with established arthritis are 79% more likely to report ADL limitations compared to those who have had arthritis for shorter duration. For each unit increase in severity of arthritis, the odds of having ADL limitations increase by 43.3%. None of the types of arthritis were significantly more or less likely to report ADL limitations compared to those with osteoarthritis.

Unlike ADL limitations, duration of arthritis is not significantly related to IADL limitations. Age is significantly related to IADL limitations, so for every year increase in age, the odds of reporting IADL limitations increase by 5.1%. Severity of arthritis is also positively related to IADL limitations, so that for each unit increase in severity of arthritis, the odds of having IADL limitations increase by 12.1%. Those with rheumatoid arthritis have 21.2% greater odds of reporting IADL limitations compared to those with

Table 2. Unstandardized Regression Coefficients Estimating the Effect of Age, Duration, Severity, and Type of Arthritis on Functional Limitations ($N = 4,903$).

	Coefficient (t-stat)
Age	0.037***
	(7.14)
Established Duration	0.759***
	(4.98)
Severity of Arthritis	0.647***
	(15.78)
Type of Arthritis[a]	
Rheumatoid	−0.093
	(−0.94)
Gout/Lupus	−0.752**
	(−2.61)
Arthritis due to an Injury	−0.157
	(−1.15)
Gender (Female)	0.668***
	(6.04)
Race (Non-whites)	0.145
	(1.07)
Marital Status (Not Married)	0.030
	(0.35)
Education	−0.100***
	(−6.02)
Household Income	−0.138***
	(−4.44)
Net Wealth	−0.048***
	(−3.5)
Insurance	0.048
	(0.21)
# of Chronic Conditions	0.537***
	(18.09)
Self-Rated Sight	−0.391***
	(−9.72)
Self-Rated Hearing	−0.193***
	(−4.23)
Participation in Physical Activity	−0.989***
	(−13.33)
BMI[b]	
Underweight	0.607
	(1.95)
Overweight	−0.032
	(−0.36)
Obese	0.641***
	(6.23)

Table 2. (*Continued*)

	Coefficient (t-stat)
Smoking Status[c]	
Current Smoker	0.340**
	(3.12)
Former Smoker	0.078
	(0.95)
R-Square	37.1

$*p<0.05$, $**p<0.01$, $***p<0.001$: two-tailed tests.
[a]Osteoarthritis = reference category.
[b]Normal weight = reference category.
[c]Never smoked = reference category.

osteoarthritis, while those with gout or lupus have 58.7% lower odds of reporting IADL limitations compared to those with osteoarthritis.

This research also confirms the independent effects of various other factors on functional limitations and disability. Females with arthritis have more functional limitations compared to males with arthritis, but do not have higher odds of reporting ADL or IADL limitations. Given that past research shows women have increased functional limitations *and* disability compared to males (Arber & Ginn, 1993; Wray & Blaum, 2001), more research is necessary to examine differences by gender in the onset of ADL and IADL limitations.

Education is negatively related to the number of functional limitations and the odds of reporting IADL limitations, but not to the odds of reporting ADL limitations. This suggests that among adults with arthritis, education matters less among those with the most severe physical functioning tasks, but does matter for less severe physical functioning tasks. Income and net wealth are important predictors of all three measures of physical functioning, which confirms the importance of income and net wealth on physical health (Link & Phelan, 1995). Research shows that income and net wealth are associated with the likelihood of remaining free from disability (Clark, Stump, Hui, & Wolinsky, 1998).

Several behavioral and health status factors are important in predicting physical functioning. As the number of chronic conditions those with arthritis experience increases, the number of functional limitations increase as well. Eyesight and hearing ability are also associated with all three outcomes. As eyesight and hearing improve, respondents report fewer functional limitations and have lower odds of reporting ADL and IADL limitations.

Table 3. Logistic Regression Estimating the Effect of Age, Duration, Severity, and Type of Arthritis on ADLs ($N = 4,927$) and IADLs ($N = 4,648$).

	Odds Ratios (t-stat)	
	ADLs	IADLs
Age	1.025***	1.051***
	(4.18)	(8.48)
Established Duration	1.790**	1.187
	(2.9)	(1.08)
Severity of Arthritis	1.433***	1.121*
	(9.59)	(2.5)
Type of Arthritis[a]		
Rheumatoid	1.047	1.212*
	(0.49)	(2)
Gout/Lupus	0.855	0.413*
	(−0.66)	(−2.26)
Arthritis due to an Injury	1.038	1.175
	(0.32)	(1.07)
Gender (Female)	1.034	0.859
	(0.36)	(−1.7)
Race (Non-whites)	1.304*	1.135
	(2.05)	(0.95)
Marital Status (Not Married)	0.886	1.133
	(−1.3)	(1.59)
Education	0.990	0.938***
	(−0.62)	(−4.22)
Household Income	0.937*	0.994*
	(−2.42)	(−0.19)
Net Wealth	0.961***	0.958***
	(−3.71)	(−3.96)
Insurance	0.839	0.933
	(−0.78)	(−0.25)
# of Chronic Conditions	1.376***	1.353***
	(11.12)	(7.8)
Self-Rated Sight	0.756***	0.784***
	(−4.92)	(−5.06)
Self-Rated Hearing	0.907*	0.863***
	(−2.03)	(−3.41)
Participation in Physical Activity	0.519***	0.523***
	(−7.09)	(−7.72)
BMI[b]		
Underweight	1.538	3.175***
	(1.26)	(4.5)
Overweight	0.970	0.877
	(−0.28)	(−1.27)
Obese	1.378*	1.166
	(2.35)	(1.21)

Table 3. (*Continued*)

	Odds Ratios (t-stat)	
	ADLs	IADLs
Smoking Status^c		
Current Smoker	1.065	1.314
	(0.51)	(1.86)
Former Smoker	0.911	1.019
	(−0.92)	(0.21)

$^*p<0.05$, $^{**}p<0.01$, $^{***}p<0.001$: two-tailed tests.
^{a}Osteoarthritis = reference category.
^{b}Normal weight = reference category.
^{c}Never smoked = reference category.

This research also confirms the importance of physical activity on physical functioning (Clark et al., 1998; Dunlop et al., 2003b). Adults with arthritis who are physically active at least 3 times per week have fewer functional limitations and have lower odds of reporting ADL and IADL limitations compared to adults with arthritis who are not physically active at least three times per week. Other research also demonstrates that moderate physical activity relieves arthritis pain and stiffness (U.S. Department of Health and Human Services, 2005). Similarly, those who are obese have more functional limitations and have higher odds of reporting ADL limitations compared to those who are normal weight, while those who are underweight have higher odds of reporting IADL limitations compared to those who are normal weight. This suggests that underweight persons with arthritis are able to perform tasks such as bathing, dressing, walking, and climbing stairs while obese persons with arthritis are not, and obese persons with arthritis are more able to do social tasks such as grocery shopping and managing money while underweight persons with arthritis are not. While the focus of this research is not the impact of BMI on physical functioning among those with arthritis, this finding is certainly interesting and deserves further investigation.

Those who smoke have more functional limitations compared to those who have never smoked. However, smoking is not associated with the odds of having ADL or IADL limitations. This suggests that smoking is an important predictor of the number of less severe limitations one experiences but not an important predictor of experiencing the onset of more severe limitations.

DISCUSSION

This research examines the impact of age, duration of arthritis, severity of arthritis, and type of arthritis on three outcomes, which are part of the disability process: functional limitations, ADL limitations, and IADL limitations. Results indicate that age and severity of arthritis are key predictors of all three outcomes for those with arthritis. The effect of duration of arthritis is only a significant predictor of functional limitations and ADL limitations. Although this finding suggests those who have lived with arthritis for a longer time will have more disability, this finding is not uniform across all outcomes. Duration of arthritis is not significantly related to IADL limitations. IADL activities are strongly linked to performing particular social roles and have less to do with physical functioning compared to the ADL tasks and functional tasks (Bruce, 2001; Clark et al., 1997; Verbrugge & Jette, 1994). There is no statistical difference between those with established duration of arthritis compared to those who have had it for a shorter duration, suggesting those with arthritis may adapt to social tasks better than to physical tasks. The support and resources that one uses to adjust to IADL limitations may be more effective over time compared to the resources used to adjust to functional limitations and ADL disability. Friends and family may be more accessible and willing to help with social tasks over time, such as grocery shopping or managing money, than with physical tasks such as bathing or getting in and out of bed. The resources available to those with disabilities, such as assistive equipment and home modifications, may be more effective in helping older adults cope with IADL limitations over time compared to the resources that assist older adults in coping with functional limitations or ADL limitations. For example, a telephone with large buttons may help older adults make telephone calls long after a person initially reports difficulty making telephone calls, yet a handrail may only help an older adult walk until they need the next level of assistance. Further research is necessary to explore why duration of arthritis is significantly related to ADL and functional limitations, yet not related to IADL limitations. Understanding social support and other resources used to cope with their physical limitations may shed light on these findings.

Those with gout or lupus have significantly fewer functional limitations and are less likely to report IADL limitations compared to those with osteoarthritis. Because those with gout or lupus often experience periods of activity or inflammation followed by periods of inactivity (remission), it is not surprising that those with gout and lupus are less likely to report functional limitations and IADL limitations. Those with rheumatoid arthritis are significantly more likely to report IADL limitations compared to those with osteoarthritis. It is surprising that those with rheumatoid arthritis are not significantly more likely to report ADL limitations. The lack of difference between the types of arthritis and osteoarthritis may be explained by the measures used to indicate type of arthritis. Each measure is not a pure indicator of only one type of arthritis and instead includes a combination of types of arthritis. While this research does provide a basis for understanding how various types of arthritis are related to the disability process, further research is needed that can compare different types of arthritis using better measures of each type of arthritis.

An important strength of this study is the ability to adjust for other determinants of functional limitations and disability such as sociodemographic factors and behavioral factors. This decreases the likelihood that confounding factors explain the association between the characteristics of arthritis and physical functioning. Results indicate that age and severity have independent effects on physical functioning. Duration is also an independent predictor of functional limitations and ADL limitations. Additionally, gender, race, education, income, net wealth, morbidity, eyesight, hearing, physical activity, BMI, and smoking status have independent effects on physical functioning. These findings confirm that physical health is not only affected by disease characteristics, but also by sociodemographic factors and behaviors. This is important when considering risk factors, interventions, and treatment.

There are several weaknesses of this research. The first involves the few number of waves utilized in constructing the duration of arthritis variable. In order to maintain an adequate sample size of respondents with arthritis, it was not possible to use data from waves prior to 1998, when the HRS original data was merged with additional subsamples. Given that arthritis is a chronic condition and many people live with it for several years, it would be beneficial to have a measure of duration that extends to time before 1998. Additionally, the sample used in this analysis does not include non-institutionalized adults. Because those in nursing homes are likely to have more functional limitations and are more disabled, excluding them from analysis likely provides underestimates of functional limitations and disability. Therefore, if non-institutionalized older adults were included in the analysis, results would likely be stronger.

Although this analysis was longitudinal, future research should consider the importance of changes in disability over time, or trajectories of disability and functional limitations. It is important to consider fluctuations in disability over time because it is possible for older adults to show declines, as well as improvement in physical functioning over time. Understanding how age, duration, severity, and type of arthritis contribute to decline and improvement in physical functioning over time may provide another layer of understanding of the relationship between arthritis and the disability process.

There is a strong need to focus on the physical functioning of older adults. Persons who are disabled may not be able to function independently. There is a general consensus that the maintenance of independence is of paramount importance to older adults. They want to remain in their own homes, have adequate self-care skills and take part in activities that they enjoy. Because arthritis is associated with functional limitations and activity limitations, many older people with arthritis are not able to maintain their independence, further decreasing their quality of life. They often need assistance from a caregiver or need to live in an assisted living or nursing home environment. Sheehan et al. (2004) suggest that with new and promising biological therapies, it is likely that difficulties in functional ability will stabilize, and ultimately result in less disability.

Because arthritis is a non-fatal condition, it is often less likely to secure research and program funding (Covinsky, 2006). However, the individual and population impacts of arthritis make it a valuable research area. Substantial increases in costs are anticipated as the US population ages and increased use is made of more costly interventions (Centers for Disease Control and Prevention, 2003). Furthermore, deteriorating physical functioning will become a large public health problem. Understanding the context of limitations may lead to improved management and support for those with functional limitations or disability. Research confirming that age, duration of arthritis, and severity of arthritis independently impact the lives of those living with arthritis can help inform public health initiatives about appropriate treatment and care and may improve the lives of millions of older adults affected by arthritis.

NOTES

1. The terms "disability" and "functional limitations" are often used inter-changeably and have been measured in various ways. For example, Johnson and Wolinsky (1993) refer to disability as basic mobility and strength tasks and refer to functional limitations as ADL and IADL tasks.

2. Because most people have zero or only a few functional limitations, and thus the distribution is highly skewed, an analysis was also conducted when the measure of functional limitations was logged. Results do not differ from the results presented in this chapter.

3. Because of possible interaction effects, interactions between age, severity, duration, and gender were tested. However, none of the interaction effects were significant and therefore are not included in the results.

REFERENCES

Arber, S., & Ginn, J. (1993). Gender and inequalities in health in later life. *Social Science and Medicine, 36*(1), 33–46.

Barlow, J. H., Cullen, L. A., & Rowe, I. F. (1999). Comparison of knowledge and psychological well-being between patients with a short disease duration (<1 year) and patients with more established rheumatoid arthritis (>10 years duration). *Patient Education and Counseling, 38*, 195–203.

Bruce, M. L. (2001). Depression and disability in late life: Directions for future research. *American Journal of Psychiatry, 9*(2), 102–112.

Centers for Disease Control and Prevention. (2003). Direct and indirect costs of arthritis and other rheumatic conditions: United States, 1997. *Morbidity and Mortality Weekly Report, 52*(46), 1124–1127.

Clark, D. O., Stump, T. E., Hui, S. L., & Wolinsky, F. D. (1998). Predictors of mobility and basic ADL difficulty among adults aged 70 years and older. *Journal of Aging and Health, 10*(4), 422–440.

Clark, D. O., Stump, T. E., & Wolinsky, F. D. (1997). A race- and gender- specific replication of five dimensions of functional limitation and disability. *Journal of Aging and Health, 9*(1), 28–42.

Covinsky, K. E. (2006). Aging, arthritis, and disability. *Arthritis and Rheumatism, 55*(2), 175–176.

Covinsky, K. E., Lindquist, K., Dunlop, D. D., Gill, T. M., & Yelin, E. H. (2008). Effect of arthritis in middle age on older-age functioning. *Journal of the American Geriatrics Society, 56*, 23–28.

Curtis, R., Groarke, A., Coughlan, R., & Gsel, A. (2004). The influence of disease severity, perceived stress, social support and coping in patients with chronic illness: A 1 year follow up. *Psychology, Health and Medicine, 9*(4), 456–475.

Curtis, R., Groarke, A., Coughlan, R., & Gsel, A. (2005). Psychological stress as a predictor of psychological adjustment and health status in patients with rheumatoid arthritis. *Patient Education and Counseling, 59*, 192–198.

Dunlop, D. D., Manheim, L. M., Song, J., & Chang, R. W. (2001). Arthritis prevalence and activity limitations in older adults. *Arthritis and Rheumatism, 44*(1), 212–221.

Dunlop, D. D., Manheim, L. M., Song, J., & Chang, R. W. (2003a). Health care utilization among older adults with arthritis. *Arthritis and Rheumatism, 49*(2), 164–171.

Dunlop, D. D., Manheim, L. M., Yelin, E. H., Song, J., & Chang, R. W. (2003b). The costs of arthritis. *Arthritis and Rheumatism, 49*(1), 101–113.

Evers, A. W. M., Kraaimaat, F. W., Geenen, R., & Bijlsma, J. W. J. (1998). Psychosocial predictors of functional change in recently diagnosed rheumatoid arthritis patients. *Behaviour Research and Therapy, 36*, 179–193.

Evers, A. W. M., Kraaimaat, F. W., Geenen, R., Jacobs, J. W. G., & Bijlsma, J. W. J. (2003). Pain coping and social support and predictors of long-term functional disability and pain in early rheumatoid arthritis. *Behaviour Research and Therapy, 41*, 1295–1310.

Fonda, S., & Herzog, A. R. (2004). *Documentation of physical functioning measured in the health and retirement study and the assess and health dynamics among the oldest old.* Survey Research Center: University of Michigan.

Fonseca, J. E., Canhao, H., Teixeira da Costa, J. C., da Silva, P., & Queiroz, M. V. (2002). Global functional status in rheumatoid arthritis: Disease durations and patient age. *Clinical Rheumatology, 21*, 32–34.

Gill, T. M., Robison, J. T., & Tinetti, M. E. (1998). Difficulty and dependence: Two components of the disability continuum among community-living older persons. *Annals of Internal Medicine, 128*, 96–101.

Hommel, K. A., Wagner, J. L., Chaney, J. M., White, M. M., & Mullins, L. L. (2004). Perceived importance of activities of daily living and arthritis helplessness in rheumatoid arthritis. *Journal of Psychosomatic Research, 57*, 159–164.

Hootman, J. M., & Helmick, C. G. (2006). Projections of US prevalence of arthritis associated activity limitations. *Arthritis and Rheumatism, 54*(1), 226–229.

Johnson, R. J., & Wolinsky, F. D. (1993). The structure of health status among older adults: Disease, disability, functional limitation, and perceived health. *Journal of Health and Social Behavior, 34*(June), 105–121.

Johnson, R. J., & Wolinsky, F. D. (1994). Gender, race, and health: The structure of health status among older adults. *The Gerontologist, 34*(1), 24–35.

Kaplan, G. A., Strawbridge, W. J., Camacho, T., & Cohen, R. D. (1993). Factors associated with change in physical functioning in the elderly: A six-year prospective study. *Journal of Aging and Health, 5*(1), 140–153.

Katz, P. (1995). The impact of rheumatoid arthritis on life activities. *Arthritis Care and Research, 8*(4), 272–278.

Kosorok, M. R., Omenn, G. S., Diehr, P., Koepsell, T. D., & Patrick, D. L. (1992). Restricted activity days among older adults. *Journal of Public Health, 82*(9), 1263–1267.

Leigh, J. P., & Fries, J. F. (1993). Tobit, fixed effects, and cohort analysis of the relationship between severity and duration of rheumatoid arthritis. *Social Science and Medicine, 36*(11), 1495–1502.

Leigh, J. P., Fries, J. F., & Parikh, N. (1992). Severity of disability and duration of disease in rheumatoid arthritis. *The Journal of Rheumatology, 19*(12), 1906–1911.

Leveille, S. G., Wee, C. C., & Iezzoni, L. I. (2005). Trends in obesity and arthritis among baby boomers. *American Journal of Public Health, 95*(9), 1607–1613.

Link, B. G., & Phelan, J. C. (1995). Social conditions as fundamental causes of disease. *Journal of Health and Social Behavior, 35*(Extra Issue), 80–94.

Long, J. S., & Pavalko, E. K. (2004). The life course of activity limitations: Exploring indicators of functional limitations over time. *Journal of Aging and Health, 16*(4), 490–516.

Meenan, R. F., Kazis, L. E., Anthony, J. M., & Wallin, B. A. (1991). The clinical and health status of patients with recent-onset rheumatoid arthritis. *Arthritis and Rheumatism, 34*, 761–765.

Nagi, S. Z. (1976). An epidemiology of disability among adults in the United States. *Milbank Memorial Fund Quarterly, 54*, 439–468.

Parker, M. G., & Thorslund, M. (2007). Health trends in the elderly population: Getting better and getting worse. *The Gerontologist, 47*(2), 150–158.

Penninx, B. W. J. H., Beekman, A. T. F., Ormel, J., Kriegsman, D. M. W., Boeke, J. P., Van Eijk, J. Th. M., & Deeg, D. J. H. (1996). Psychological status among elderly people with chronic diseases: Does type of disease play a part? *Journal of Psychosomatic Research*, *40*(5), 521–534.

Rosow, I., & Breslau, N. (1966). A guttman health scale for the aged. *Journal of Gerontology*, *21*, 556–559.

Serbo, B., & Jajic, I. (1991). Relationship of the functional status, duration of the disease and pain intensity and some psychological variables in patients with rheumatoid arthritis. *Clinical Rheumatology*, *10*(4), 419–422.

Sheehan, T. J., DuBrava, S., Fifield, J., Reisine, S., & DeChello, L. (2004). Rate of change in functional limitations for patients with rheumatoid arthritis: Effects of sex, age, and duration of illness. *The Journal of Rheumatology*, *31*(7), 1286–1292.

StataCorp. (2005). *Stata statistical software: Release 9*. College Station, TX: StataCorp LP.

Treharne, G. J., Kitas, G. D., Lyons, A. C., & Booth, D. A. (2005). Well-being in rheumatoid arthritis: The effects of disease duration and psychosocial factors. *Journal of Health Psychology*, *10*(3), 457–474.

Treharne, G. J., Lyons, A. C., Booth, D. A., Mason, S. R., & Kitas, G. D. (2004). Reactions to disability in patients with early versus established rheumatoid arthritis. *Scandinavian Journal of Rheumatology*, *33*, 30–38.

U.S. Department of Health and Human Services. (2005). *Preventing chronic diseases: Investing wisely in health. Preventing arthritis pain*. Atlanta, GA: U.S. Department of Health and Human Services, National Center for Chronic Disease Prevention and Health Promotion, Centers for Disease Control and Prevention. Retrieved on May, 2008, from http://www.cdc.gov/nccdphp/publications/factsheets/Prevention/pdf/arthritis.pdf

Verbrugge, L. M. (1992). Disability transitions for older persons with arthritis. *Journal of Aging and Health*, *4*(2), 212–243.

Verbrugge, L. M., & Jette, A. M. (1994). The disablement process. *Social Science and Medicine*, *38*(1), 1–14.

Verbrugge, L. M., & Juarez, L. (2001). Profile of arthritis disability. *Public Health Reports*, *116*(Suppl.), 157–179.

Verbrugge, L. M., & Patrick, D. L. (1995). Seven chronic conditions: Their impact on US adults' activity levels and use of medical services. *American Journal of Public Health*, *85*(2), 173–182.

Vradenburg, J. A., Simoes, E. J., Jackson-Thompson, J., & Murayi, T. (2002). The prevalence of arthritis and activity limitations and their predictors in Missouri. *Journal of Community Health*, *27*(2), 91–107.

Wolfe, F. (2000). A reappraisal of HAQ disability in rheumatoid arthritis. *Arthritis Rheumatology*, *43*, 2751–2761.

Wray, L. A., & Blaum, C. S. (2001). Explaining the role of sex on disability: A population-based study. *The Gerontologist*, *41*(4), 499–510.

Yelin, E. H. (1992). Arthritis. The cumulative impact of a common chronic condition. *Arthritis Rheumatology*, *35*(5), 489–497.

Yelin, E. H., Lubeck, D., Holman, H., & Epstein, W. (1987). The impact of rheumatoid arthritis and osteoarthritis: The activities of patients with rheumatoid arthritis and osteoarthritis compared to controls. *Journal of Rheumatology*, *14*, 710–717.

Zimmer, Z., Hickey, T., & Searle, M. S. (1997). The pattern of change in leisure activity behavior among older adults with arthritis. *The Gerontologist*, *37*(3), 384–392.

WEIGHT LOSS SURGERY PATIENTS' NEGOTIATIONS OF MEDICINE'S INSTITUTIONAL LOGIC ☆

Patricia Drew

ABSTRACT

In this chapter I explore how conflicting discursive claims made by the medical community are consequential for bariatric weight loss surgery patients. Bariatric surgery has become increasingly common in the United States since the 1990s, with over 177,000 Americans undergoing surgery in 2006. Despite the surgery's growing popularity, the US medical community does not wholeheartedly endorse the surgery. Rather, different members of the medical community espouse contradictory evaluations of weight loss surgery. I broadly characterize this intra-medical community controversy and, then, discuss how conflicting claims have helped shape the bariatric surgery industry's discursive conception of an "ideal patient." Next, I analyze actual patients' negotiations of the ideal patient

---

☆ An earlier version of this paper was presented with Denise D. Bielby (bielbyd@soc.ucsb.edu) at the Annual Meetings of the American Sociological Association, New York, NY, August 10–14, 2007.

Care for Major Health Problems and Population Health Concerns: Impacts on Patients, Providers and Policy
Research in the Sociology of Health Care, Volume 26, 65–92
Copyright © 2008 by Emerald Group Publishing Limited
All rights of reproduction in any form reserved
ISSN: 0275-4959/doi:10.1016/S0275-4959(08)26004-7

archetype, and find that patients' responses follow three paths: embracing the ideal, having a mixed response to the ideal, and strategically complying with the ideal. As patients are compelled to grapple with the ideal archetype in order to access surgery, I conclude that the ideal archetype acts as a discursive frame connecting individual patients to broad bariatric surgery discourses.

INTRODUCTION

Bariatric surgery, more commonly known as weight loss surgery, is an increasingly common procedure that causes morbidly obese patients to lose significant weight. People often lose 100 or more pounds in the year following surgery. Over 177,000 Americans underwent weight loss surgery in 2006, an increase of over 800% since 1995 [American Society for Metabolic and Bariatric Surgery (ASMBS), 2007a]. While many sociological studies have examined and problematized fatness and obesity in recent years (cf, Monaghan, 2006; Oliver, 2006; Rich & Evans, 2005; Saguy & Riley, 2005), researchers have only begun to investigate the obesity surgery phenomenon. Natalie Boero (2007) and Julie Ferris (2003) both briefly mention weight loss surgery in their analysis of the media's obesity framing. Talya Salant and Heena Santry (2006) analyzed differences in Internet marketing strategies for weight loss surgery between university and private hospitals. Leanne Joanisse (2005) and Karen Throsby (2006) found that the surgery experience transforms patients' identities. Throsby (2007) has further asserted that bariatric patients account for their fatness by utilizing popular discourses, for example, stating that they had a "fat gene." None of these studies, however, have examined medical community discussions about weight loss surgery, nor have they demonstrated how surgery patients understand and reflect upon this medical information.

While an actual bariatric procedure may take only a few hours, pre-surgical preparations can take months or years. In order to have surgery, patients must go through a battery of physiological exams, gain authorization from their surgeon and, typically, their insurance company. Frequently, patients must also diet, join support groups, and meet with affiliated staff such as nutritionists, psychologists, and physical therapists. Bariatric surgery is clearly a lengthy and involved process. In this chapter, I examine medical debates about bariatric surgery, and how these debates have resulted in the construction of what I term "ideal patient" guidelines that influence patients' adaptation to surgically induced weight loss. Specifically, I explore how actual patients negotiate these patient guidelines.

THEORETICAL CONSIDERATIONS

The public often considers obesity to be unattractive (Bordo, 1993; Stinson, 2001), a sign of laziness or sloth (Evans, 2006), an outcome of corporate greed (Nestle, 2002), and/or a cause of rising public health costs [World Health Organization (WHO), 1999]. Researchers and policymakers often adopt these negative assessments (cf, Thompson, 2001). More rarely, scholars, activists, and the public view obesity as an appropriate body size which has been wrongfully demonized (Gimlin, 2002; Wann, 1998). Social and policy discussions are infused with moral debates about obesity's costs, ethical dimensions, and individuals' personal responsibility for their body size (Throsby, 2007).

The obese body does not merely represent an ethical conundrum. Obesity is also simultaneously viewed as a medical condition. In medical literature, obese bodies are routinely depicted as unhealthy (Kushner, 2003); obesity is portrayed as causing co-morbidity conditions such as sleep apnea, diabetes, and cardiovascular problems (*ibid*); and obesity is increasingly described as a physical manifestation of a psychological problem (Joranby, Pineda, & Gold, 2005). The US government has long problematized obesity, and in 2004 Medicare classified obesity as a disease [United States Department of Health and Human Services (HHS), 2004]. The medically oriented term "obesity epidemic" has been appropriated by health policy organizations such as the Centers for Disease Control (1999), the National Institutes of Health (2004) and the World Health Organization (1999), as well as the medical community and popular media. Together, these depictions reveal the medicalization of obesity; that is, obesity has come to be "defined in terms of health or illness" (Riessman, 1983). The medical conceptualization of obesity implies subsequent medical treatment and oversight (*ibid*; Conrad & Schneider, 1980). Bariatric surgery is clearly an outgrowth of obesity's medicalization, as the surgery is considered a solution for obesity and its related health conditions.

With this study I am specifically interested in examining the influence of the medical community's discursive depictions of bariatric surgery. Medical messages are particularly significant because surgeons regulate patients' obesity surgery access. In order to examine the connection

between medical messages and patients' understandings of their health care experiences,
I draw upon discourse and framing literatures as well as insights from the field of narrative studies. I view "discourses" as the language and discussions that emerge surrounding a phenomenon (Foucault, 1969). I utilize Julianne Cheek's (2004, p. 1142) assertion that "a discourse consists of a set of common assumptions that sometimes, indeed often, may be so taken for granted as to be invisible or assumed.". Erving Goffman's (1974) concept of "frames" compliments this definition; he views frames as organizational tools which arrange experiences, perceptions, and views. Individuals, social groups, social institutions, and loose cultural constituencies all engage in framing; the frames they create propose ways of understanding or comprehending phenomena (ibid). Or, as Goffman-inspired scholars Christine Everingham, Heading, and Linda (2006) state, "[How] a situation is understood depends upon how the experience is organized – what principles of social organization come into play" (p. 1746).

Discursive frames both directly and indirectly shape discussions about social issues and, thus, are consequential for individual. They help to shape people's comprehensions of phenomena and limit/permit responses. James Holstein and Jaber Gubrium (2000) refer to this activity as "interpretive practice," where situated people replicate, respond to, and transform discourses. I draw upon this characterization to study the relationship between medical messages and individual patients' interpretations of and responses to these messages.

Narrative researchers assert that social discourses appear within individuals' narratives (Charmaz, 1994; Collins, 2003; Gimlin, 2007). Such studies suggest that people selectively incorporate information from prevailing social discourses into their self-stories. Further, narrative scholars argue that available social scripts and schemas help to shape individuals' self conceptions (Lawler, 2002; Mason, 2002; Matthews Lovering, 1995). The lengthy and intensive process of weight loss surgery can be a significant experience for patients to reflect upon and incorporate into their self-narratives. At the present, researchers have not sufficiently explored how individuals utilize discourses and frames within their self-narratives. I intend to clarify the connection between discourse and framing studies and narrative studies by, first, demonstrating how bariatric weight loss surgery debates have shaped surgical discourse and, next, showing how patients' grapple with surgical discourses in their personal narratives.

METHODS

The field of bariatric surgery is not without controversy, even within the medical community, and in order to qualitatively explore the relationship between these medical debates and personal conceptions, I have collected data from both medical sources and weight loss surgery patients through interviews and surveys.[1]

Data concerning patients' bariatric surgery experiences comes from interviews and surveys gathered between December 2005 and October 2006. Participants were primarily recruited through an announcement in a large, nationwide bariatric information website. Fifty-five filled out an open-ended survey, 41 were interviewed via telephone interview, and 3 were interviewed in-person. Respondents came from 34 states. Eighty-three respondents were post-operative and 16 respondents were pre-operative at the time of research participation. The mean age was 42. Ninety (90%) of my respondents were women; 65% of respondents were self-identified white women. In total, 74 respondents identified their race as white, 17 did not state their race, and 8 stated that they were a race other than white: three were African American; three identified as Latina, one person identified as half-Asian/half white, and one person identified as Native American.

My sample resembles the population of US weight loss surgery patients in several categories. The Nationwide Inpatient Sample (NIS), the largest all-payer inpatient database in the US, indicates that the mean age for bariatric surgery patients in 2002 was 41.7 and women comprised 84% of surgical patients (Santry, Gillen, & Lauderdale, 2005). The study was unable to report the surgical population's racial composition, as over 20% of the NIS data was missing information on racial background.

In order to examine how individuals interpret and respond to medical discourses, I utilize narrative interview analysis, an approach that views respondents' interview data as representative of their worldviews (Silverman, 2000). The use of personal narratives has been found to be important to the construction of individuals' self-concept and in identity formation (Shelton & Johnson, 2006). I analyzed interview and survey data by examining how individuals' spoke or wrote about their medical experiences. All respondents' names have been replaced with pseudonyms.

In order to examine prominent medical weight loss surgery discourses, I gathered information from a wide array of sources. These sources include: generalist medical journals such as the *Journal of the American Medical Association*; bariatric specialty medical journals such as *Surgery for Obesity and Related Disorders*, media coverage of medical debates in the *New York*

Times and on the *Public Broadcasting System*; the pro-bariatric surgery periodical *Obesity Help*; websites of bariatric surgeons; and websites of bariatric surgery critics. I also collected government documents such as the 1978 and 1991 National Institutes of Health (NIH) Consensus Statements on Bariatric Surgery and examined statements about bariatric surgery featured on government websites, including websites of the NIH, the Centers for Disease Control, and the Food and Drug Administration. Additionally, I conducted an interview with a senior manager of a national health insurance association regarding infighting among bariatric surgeons' associations.

I repeatedly examined medical and government materials using qualitative content analysis, a method that concentrates upon analyzing the substance of a document and then recording and analyzing the associated meanings (Altheide, 1996). I analyzed the materials for the presence and content of obesity surgery discourses. Discourses were apparent when physicians, surgeons, or other medical actors would make statements and express views about bariatric surgery.

DEVELOPING AN IDEAL PATIENT ARCHETYPE

Historical and current bariatric surgery debates have helped to shape present-day patient guidelines. Accordingly, in order to understand the development of the ideal patient archetype, with which patients are compelled to comply, it is necessary to understand bariatric surgery's history. Weight loss surgery was initially developed in 1954 with the advent of the jejunoileal bypass. This operation promoted weight loss by circumventing most of the intestinal track and, thus, limited the calories absorbed by the body. Patients lost vast amounts of weight, but many experienced side effects such as constant diarrhea, malnutrition, and the toxic overgrowth of bacteria in the bypassed intestine (Griffen, Bivins, & Bell, 1983). The controversial procedure used in early practice was largely discontinued by the 1970s and was severely critiqued by the NIH in 1978. The bariatric field had similarly limited success with other procedures including gastroplasty (aka "stomach stapling") in the 1970s and biliopancreatic diversion in the 1980s; each operation initially held promise yet later revealed negative side effects.

Despite the development of new surgical procedures such as gastric bypass and the Lap-Band, and regardless of a 1991 NIH statement endorsing high-quality surgery, the dangerous reputation of earlier procedures has continued to taint medical opinion. Medical critics have questioned the surgery's safety, noting that 40% of patients experience some type of complication within 6 months of surgery (Encinosa, Bernard, Chen, & Steiner, 2006; Zingmond, McGory, & Ko, 2005). Critics – including some bariatric surgeons – also question whether all surgeons are well trained (Flum et al., 2005). Other skeptics ask if hospitals are overly motivated by potential profit when soliciting patients (Grady, 2004). Medical community skeptics associated with the activist organization National Association for the Advancement of Fat Acceptance and Health at Every Size question the connection between obesity and health, arguing that sedentary thin people are often less healthy than active obese people (Goldberg, 1996).

Bariatric supporters within the medical community, including many bariatric surgeons, surgeons' professional organizations, and for-profit and not-for-profit bariatric industry affiliates, have attempted to address skeptics' criticisms while concurrently promoting obesity surgery. Proponents argue that morbid obesity causes poor health, especially chronic conditions like sleep apnea, diabetes, and hypertension [American College of Surgeons (ACS), 2007]. Supporters claim that diets do not work and that surgery is the only viable cure for morbid obesity (*ibid*). Furthermore, supporters argue that bariatric surgery can "provide previously unimaginable full remission" [Surgical Review Corporation (SRC), 2007] of health problems. Moreover, bariatric supporters assert that it is important to develop measurable standards of care, and two leading professional associations, the American Society for Metabolic and Bariatric Surgery (ASMBS) and the American College of Surgeons (ACS), have each set up benchmarks for best-practices.

The ASMBS[2] is the largest bariatrics association in the US with over 3,100 members (ASMBS, 2007b). The organization holds annual conferences and publishes its own medical journal. In 2004 the ASMBS created the Centers of Excellence (COE) accreditation program. This program evaluates hospitals, surgeons, and surgical groups performing weight loss surgery; those that meet benchmarks are recognized. The other leading pro-bariatric organization is the ACS, which has over 70,000 members. Unlike the ASMBS, the ACS is not solely dedicated to bariatric surgery; rather, it reviews and monitors hospitals through its Bariatric Surgery Center Network (BSCN) accreditation program. As with the COE program, the BSCN recognizes hospitals that meet its standards. The ASMBS, the ACS, and their accreditation programs have become the preeminent voices of the bariatric surgery field. As these associations have grown in significance, their standards for patient selection and patient care have influenced policies and trends throughout the bariatric surgery industry.

I have found that the emphasis placed upon accreditation is one way that bariatric supporters control weight loss surgery discourse. Through this framing, pro-bariatrics move conversation from "Is the surgery appropriate?" to "Under what conditions is the surgery appropriate?" Consequently, this discursive shift aims to redefine the terms of the surgery debate. Central to how medical discourse about surgical weight loss becomes influential is that, as accreditation program have become more prevalent, insurers have often turned to these organizations to establish and regulate quality criteria. Some insurers cover patient claims only from approved centers. Correspondingly, hospitals and surgeons view program participation as both financially beneficial and admirable (Guadagnino, 2007). By 2007, 307 hospitals or surgical groups, and 540 surgeons belonged to at least one of the accreditation programs, many belonged to both (ACS, 2007; ASMBS, 2007).

As accreditation programs have grown swiftly in popularity and have successfully positioned themselves as industry leaders, their certification guidelines have helped to determine current bariatric practices and care standards. These guidelines also address concerns of skeptics within the medical community that unprepared hospitals and surgeons are entering the bariatric market primarily for profit. For instance, surgeons must demonstrate their expertise and dedication by performing at least 125 surgeries prior to accreditation qualification. Surgeons must then perform at least 50 surgeries annually to maintain certification. For hospitals to gain bariatric surgery accreditation they must perform at least 150 surgeries annually. Accreditation programs also set standards for hospitals to be staffed and equipped sufficiently to care for morbidly obese patients (ACS, 2007; SRC, 2007).

Most significant for understanding patients' bariatric surgery experiences, the accreditation process emphasizes patient attributes as a way of ensuring high-quality surgery outcomes. According to ASMBS and ACS guidelines, patients are required to meet minimum weight and health criteria; they should also have a verifiable history of dieting attempts. Patients are required to give informed consent. This involves extensive education about the surgical procedure and information about the lifestyle changes required (ACS, 2007; SRC, 2007). These patient selection principles are designed to promote high-quality care and also address critics' concerns that surgeons are inappropriately persuading prospective patients to undergo surgery.

Accreditation guidelines, then, matter for patients as well as for the bariatric industry.

The parallel development of the ASMBS and ACS accreditation programs is however, fraught with inter-organizational competition. According to a health insurance association senior manager who has worked closely with officials from both organizations, the ASMBS and ACS are "fighting tooth and nail" to be in control of bariatric standards (interview March 22, 2007). The ASMBS leadership asserts that the older, more established ACS is trying to position itself as the central bariatric authority. The ACS claims that the ASMBS is "self-serving and trying to promote surgery" by garishly increasing publicity (*ibid*). While these organizational disputes do not directly focus on the role of the patient, these squabbles and the existence of competing programs have increased attention to the standards for hospital accreditation for practice of the surgery. In short, as patient selection and compliance have become more central components of certification, actual patients have been increasingly impacted by the presence of the criteria comprising accreditation.

Both the ASMBS and ACS have drawn upon a 1991 National Institutes of Health (NIH) Consensus Statement in determining who is an appropriate surgery candidate. The competitive development of the ASMBS and ACS accreditation programs was a key component in the bariatric industry's increased adoption and utilization of NIH standards. Prior to the creation of the ASMBS and ACS programs, the NIH criteria were not consistently utilized throughout the bariatric industry. This statement has been a touchstone for pro-bariatrics as it indicates "official" government validation of weight loss surgery. As such, it is an essential component to the medical discourse that frames patient knowledge and understanding of surgical weight loss procedures. Ultimately, the NIH guidelines shape patients' eligibility, frame patients' self-understandings, and influence the meaning and significance of patients' experiences with the procedure.

Upon reviewing the NIH guidelines and comparing them with the requirements of accreditation programs and respondents' reports of their surgeons' requirements, I have identified four components of an ideal patient archetype. While individual surgeons and surgical practices create their own patient policies, all of my respondents indicated that their surgeons incorporated at least some aspects of the ideal patient archetype. Most surgical practices, then, are best described as implementing variants of the ideal patient archetype. By exploring the ideal patient criteria we can see how bariatric supporters frame the weight loss surgery discourse and how this frame influences patients' experiences.

The first ideal patient characteristic, *appropriate physiology*, outlines weight and health criteria. According to the NIH, patients should have a BMI (body mass index) of 40 or more; that is, they should be approximately 100 pounds (or more) overweight.[3] Patients with a BMI between 35 and 40 (roughly 70–100 pounds overweight) may be considered for surgery if they suffer from related health conditions, often called co-morbid conditions or comorbidities. Pro-bariatric organizations and individual surgeons frequently use the NIH physiology guidelines. For example, association websites and individual surgeon sites, accreditation program manuals, and the patients I interviewed repeated these guidelines. Bariatric surgery organizations and providers often conceptualized patients who meet BMI and comorbidity requirements as diseased.

In the second aspect of the ideal patient archetype, prospective patients are encouraged to demonstrate an *appropriate diet history*. The NIH expected prospective patients to be dieters, but unsuccessful dieters. The accreditation programs each suggest that patients have a documented dieting history, and many insurers require all patients to have a 6-month documented dieting history. This criterion is also frequently implemented in surgeons' offices. Some individual surgeons permit patients to submit previous, recorded dieting attempts such as personal food diaries or records from commercial weight loss centers such as Weight Watchers. Others require patients to initiate a new diet through the bariatric surgeon or their primary care physician. Many surgeons also require patients to undergo an additional diet in the month prior to surgery. Patients could only have surgery when these pre-surgical diets were complete.

The third aspect of the ideal patient archetype, *appropriate behavior*, details patients' willingness to follow surgical instructions, become educated about the surgery, and participate in pre- and post-surgical care. The NIH recommends that prospective patients be evaluated by a "multidisciplinary team with access to medical, surgical, psychiatric, and nutritional expertise" (1991, p. 12). Patients are expected to willingly see all of these experts as well as comply with the experts' particular requests, whether that is to undergo therapy or to lose weight before surgery. The ASMBS and ACS appropriate NIH criteria by mandating the following practices: certified centers must provide diet and exercise counseling, psychological counseling, plastic surgery consultations, and life-long follow-up care. Consistent with these directives, I found that almost all of my respondents were required to meet with a wide variety of experts before and after surgery. Typically patients first attended a large orientation meeting sponsored by the surgeon or hospital. At this meeting, one or more surgeons gave a lecture about the surgical procedure, physiological requirements, and the pre- and post-operative behavioral requirements. Sometimes former patients also spoke about their surgery experiences. Prospective patients were only allowed to make an appointment with the bariatric surgeon after attending the orientation meeting, and typically a staff member was at the meeting to make sure they signed in.

After the surgeon and patient met and consulted about the patient's case, the surgical staff set up additional patient appointments. Some were physiological exams, for instance, tests with a cardiologist. Other appointments included discussions of pre- and post-surgical diets with nutritionists and psychological screening with psychologists or psychiatrists. Most respondents reported being asked or told to attend surgeon-sponsored support groups both before and after surgery. Some of these groups were led by social workers and other groups were led by post-operative patients.

The fourth and final aspect of the ideal patient archetype is *appropriate attitude*, which governed the patient's motivation, mental approach to surgery, and proper desire for surgery. The NIH recommends that patients should "strongly desire substantial weight loss," be "well informed and motivated," and have a "clear and realistic understanding of how their lives may change after surgery (*ibid*, p. 8). Thus, the appropriate patient attitude put forth by bariatric supporters promotes an ideal patient that wants weight loss surgery, but not *too* much. Patients are expected to be both desirous for the surgery and "realistic" about surgical risks. Individual surgeons implement the appropriate attitude theme in multiple ways. First, at a patient's initial meeting with the bariatric surgeon, some respondents reported that they were required to demonstrate their knowledge about what the surgery was, how laparoscopic surgery was different than open surgery, and how they need to change their diet and exercise habits after surgery. For surgeons, these quizzes indicated how seriously the patient was approaching obesity surgery and whether or not the patient was appropriately reflecting on their obesity as a medical condition. Patients were also required to demonstrate their tempered, reasonable expectations to medical staff and to psychologists. If prospective patients discussed weight loss surgery as an easy obesity cure, surgeons were likely to dismiss their case or provide them with more education about appropriate post-surgical behaviors. In this way, patients not only had to engage in proper behaviors, but they had to approach those behaviors with the correct attitude.

Perhaps the most revealing demonstration of surgery providers' perspective regarding appropriate patient attitude is providers' assertion that patients accept surgery as a "tool." Surgeons and surgical staff frequently use the tool metaphor; it has also been appropriated by pro-bariatric periodicals, makers of bariatric products, and online support groups. When weight loss surgery is portrayed as a tool, it is seen as a device that enables patients to lose weight they would otherwise be unable to lose. To underscore the notion of the surgery as a tool is the surgeons' expectation that patients' grasp that this surgical tool will not work, however, without patients' constant participation and oversight. Consequently, and often linked to the tool metaphor, patients are also encouraged to think of their surgery as a discrete aspect of a larger weight loss "journey." Providers encourage patients to view their weight loss as an ongoing, life-transforming experience. Providers claim the bariatric journey never ends, and imply that patients must constantly monitor themselves to make sure that they are journeying in the appropriate, slimmer direction. Surgeons and their staff strongly imply that patients must vigilantly monitor themselves and patient success is presented as if it depended upon individuals' willingness to accept responsibility for their bodies. Patients were expected to assume the attitude that they were ultimately responsible for their actions and monitoring their feelings. While the surgical tool remained the crucial component of the weight loss journey, patients retained responsibility for the successful management of their bodies.

In sum, the different elements of physiology, diet history, behavior, and attitude are all components of the ideal patient frame. Patients become aware of this frame, and of the bariatric industry's underlying expectation that they should match the ideal criteria as they enter into the surgery process. The actual process of patient adaptation to the discursive ideal takes considerable adjustment on patients' part, and I have found that individuals vary considerably in their alignment to the patient ideal.

PATIENTS' NEGOTIATIONS OF THE IDEAL ARCHETYPE

In the following sections, I explore how actual patients understand and respond to the discursive conception of the ideal patient. I found patients negotiate the ideal archetype in three central ways. Much like Max Weber's (1949) "ideal types" these categories somewhat artificially classify individuals' idiosyncratic viewpoints; however, these categories represent the range of individuals' responses to patient guidelines. The first manner in which patients react to the ideal patient archetype is to *embrace* ideal patient attributes; 65 out of 99 respondents indicate accepting or supporting the ideal. Eighteen patients describe their responses to the ideal as *mixed*; they agree with some aspects of the ideal, but are critical of other aspects. Finally, three patients characterize their response to the ideal as *strategic*; that is, they strategically appeared to accept the ideal archetype in order to access surgery. Together, these three separate categories reveal the spectrum of patients' archetype negotiations.[4]

Thirteen open-ended survey respondents did not include enough information in their survey responses to indicate how they negotiated the ideal patient archetype. These respondents either left questions unanswered and/or listed bariatric activities they engaged in without revealing their feelings about these activities.

All of the respondents stated that they learned about bariatric program policies, including components of the ideal archetype, as they became bariatric patients. Patients became familiar with surgical guidelines and ideals as they went to bariatric medical appointments, attended orientation meetings and support group meetings, researched bariatric surgery, and chatted on online bariatric websites. The process of learning about the ideal patient archetype, then, largely occurred at the same time that individuals were becoming patients. While many patients reported that they were familiar with weight loss surgery or had independently researched surgery before contacting bariatric programs, no respondents were completely familiar with surgical guidelines before becoming bariatric surgery patients.

Embracing the Ideal

The majority of respondents embrace the ideal patient archetype, with interest levels ranging from straightforward acceptance to considerable enthusiasm. The 65 research participants who adopted the ideal patient archetype describe the ideal criteria in largely positive terms. As *embracers*, they indicate having considerable faith in bariatric guidelines and believe that their personal success is linked to their ability to abide by medical recommendations. Embracers validate physiological guidelines, willingly fulfill dieting requirements and abide by behavioral expectations. Embracers take on the ideal attitude by approaching their surgeries seriously and claiming personal responsibility for their post-surgical weight loss. Throughout their narratives, embracers are respectful of medical guidelines; they believe that guidelines are almost unfalteringly good and were put in place to ensure patient success. They are also likely to express positive sentiments about bariatric surgeons and affiliated healthcare support teams.

Embracers' acceptance of the ideal patient archetype is seen in their discussions of the four ideal patient components. For instance, embracers believe that the physiological guidelines for BMI and comorbidities are valid patient selection criteria. This is seen in the following interview excerpt, where Donna, 32, was originally dismayed to find that she didn't qualify for surgery.

> Donna: "I was initially denied by the surgeon because she said my BMI wasn't high enough. And I was really disappointed. But then, in going back and looking over copies of the paperwork that had been submitted, I discovered that a nurse had made an error and had recorded my height wrong. She had put me down as being a couple of inches taller than I actually am and...."

> Patricia: "Oh, gosh, that totally affects it."

> Donna: "Exactly. I went back to my primary care physician and I was like 'Cindy, hey!' And she looked at me and she was like, 'Oh my goodness. Let's resubmit all of this.' So we resubmitted everything and ... I got a call about a month later saying, 'Come on in. Let's do our orientation meeting.'"

As someone who accepts medical guidelines, Donna never questioned the appropriateness of her surgeon's physiological criteria. She did not criticize or dismiss medical guidelines when she was undergoing surgery prerequisites. Like other embracers, Donna was pleased that her body fit the legitimate surgery guidelines.

In a similar vein, embracers' narratives demonstrate how they came to believe that their bodies required surgical treatment. That is, embracers not only accept the medical community's physiological guidelines, they also view bariatric surgery as the necessary intervention. This realization often occurred as embracers became familiar with physiological requirements. Ed, 50, had been overweight throughout his life, but never thought that he required medical intervention.

> Ed: "It was just something that I was going to have to deal with ... I just considered that I was raised with really crappy nutritional programming from an early age, and between that and a metabolic propensity for keeping weight on anyway ..."

However, after Ed had an accident, he gained 120 pounds and began experiencing health problems. Ed's wife was intrigued by bariatric surgery, and he first heard about surgery from her. As he entered a bariatric surgery program, he redefined his body as requiring surgery. Ed then reframed his body as medically problematic, and aimed to "get rid of the comorbidities" by undergoing surgery. He uses the vernacular of the bariatric field when describing why he needs surgical intervention: "My comorbidities are sleep apnea, hypertension, hyperlipidemia, which is mainly more high triglycerides and cholesterol ..." Ed's use of medical jargon, which is similar to other embracers, suggests that embracers internalize physiological components of the ideal archetype.

Embracers additionally view their surgeons' pre-surgical dieting requirements as legitimate. Notably, when respondents talk about pre-surgical diets, they cite widely varying diet rationale. Some patients state that a dieting history is necessary to ensure that patients can commit to modifying eating habits, while others argue that diets in the month prior to surgery reduce liver size and/or liver fattiness and, thus, reduce surgical risk. The thread tying these seemingly distinct embracers together is their shared belief in their own surgeons' expertise. As embracers, these patients accept their surgeons' instructions without questions or criticisms. By believing in the unquestionable authority of their own surgeons, these patients embrace the ideal guidelines. Embracers' agreement with medical authority is seen in interview excerpts with Linda, 40, and Emma, 38.

> Linda: "I lost 38 [pounds] before my surgery. My surgeon requested that you lose at least 30 [pounds] before surgery to show that you really have the determination for the life-changing, lifestyle change."

> Emma: "They want you to lose 10 to 20 pounds before surgery so that it will shrink your liver. And the reason they want to do that is because they're going to do this with the [laparoscope]. And if your liver is not small enough, it might be harder, and they might have to open you up. ... So the day I started the diet I was 256 pounds. On the day of my surgery I was 241 pounds. ... Because I didn't cheat on this diet."

Linda and Emma draw upon different rationale when talking about pre-surgical diets. As embracers, both women believe that the medical instructions she received signify the correct and appropriate course of action. Both women take their dieting instructions seriously, indicating subscription to the ideal archetype.

Embracers similarly assert that it is crucial to comply with surgeons' behavioral requirements. For example, Kara, 38, found mandated support groups and informational seminars invaluable. She says, "I barely missed one. ... Yeah. I educated myself a lot through those meetings." Like most research participants, Kara was also required to undergo extensive physiological testing. These tests included a stress test, a cardiogram, an EKG, a few breathing tests, a sleep apnea test, an abdominal ultrasound, and blood tests. As Kara embraces the ideal patient archetype, she found all of these medical appointments worthwhile. Indeed, she believes that her successful weight loss stems from the testing she endured and the support groups she attended.

When surgeons ask embracers to undergo psychological evaluations, embracers perceive the request to be legitimate and appropriate, and willingly comply. Ed says, "Oh yeah – everybody has to do a psych eval. If you've got someone who doesn't do a psych eval, you need to call and report their surgeon to some board." Using pro-bariatric language, Ed supports the need for psychological screening, saying that he believes some patients are trying to "change something about themselves that is actually emotional rather than physical." Embracers indicate their subscription to the medical ideal when agreeing that psychological examinations are a necessary screening device.

By undergoing extensive testing, passing psychological examinations, and attending required support groups, patients who embrace the ideal archetype understand their compliance as evidence that they are having surgery for the "right" reasons. They are also likely to link their appropriate behaviors to their appropriate attitude. Embracers cite personal sacrifices and behavior modifications as evidence that they are approaching surgery properly: Emma, a "Mountain Dew junkie" and a smoker before signing up for bariatric surgery, willingly gave up both of these "vices" as she "made the commitment." She says, "I am not looking for a miracle cure. I am looking to get healthy." Similarly, other embracers assert that weight loss surgery requires self-discipline. They feel that their ability to control their bodies and their eating habits leads to permanent weight loss. Embracers thus validate the ideal patient archetype by arguing that having the right attitude is key to their success. Embracers often discuss their surgeries as a tool for weight loss rather than an obesity cure, and, therefore, understand their surgeries as a mechanism to help them combat overeating. Emma stresses the importance of respecting her surgical tool.

> Emma: "And, you know, I did not go into this lightly, and my tool is a tool, and I'm not going to abuse it, I'm not going to forget about it. And the one question I get a lot is, 'Do you ever wish that you could reverse it for a day and just eat whatever you wanted?' No."

When casting weight loss surgery as a tool that helps her to control eating patterns, Emma views herself as responsible for overseeing her surgery. Emma feels that her surgeon has done his part, and she believes that she is now ultimately responsible for using her tool correctly in order to ensure her surgical success. Like Emma, many embracers describe the post-surgical implementation of their tool as a self-directed journey from obesity to slenderness. These patients appropriated and subscribed to the ideal patient vernacular.

In sum, respondents who embrace the ideal patient archetype feel that medical guidelines for patients are useful and legitimate. They define surgical success as the ability to abide by their surgeons' medical guidelines. With one exception, all of these patients evaluate their surgical experiences positively and feel that they have done a good job fulfilling all medical criteria. By positively evaluating ideal archetype components, and by altering their own behaviors and attitudes to be in alignment with the ideal, these patients take their bodies seriously in ways suggested by the bariatric industry. However, other patients did not wholly embrace the ideal, as I describe next.

Having a Mixed Response to the Ideal

Many participants indicate that they do not completely subscribe to the ideal patient archetype. The 18 respondents with a mixed or ambivalent reaction to the ideal archetype feel that following some of the surgical guidelines is worthwhile and would lead to successful post-surgical weight loss. They simultaneously identify other components of the archetype as insignificant or as bureaucratic. The program elements defined positively and negatively varied among this *mixed responder* group. There is no ideal patient characteristic that all mixed responders validate. Similarly, there is no single characteristic that all mixed responders dismiss. For example, one mixed responder might validate attitude and behavior aspects of the ideal patient archetype while concurrently rejecting physiological and diet history components. Regardless of which elements are accepted and rejected, all mixed responders indicate ambivalence toward at least one aspect of ideal patient criteria. By selectively accepting and rejecting different ideal patient aspects, these respondents reveal ambivalence about patient guidelines that comprise the ideal archetype.

Selective agreement with elements of the ideal archetype is apparent in the narratives of the mixed responders. For instance, Bea, 52, is quick to validate physiological guidelines for patient selection. She identifies her pre-surgical BMI as severely problematic. Bea believes that diabetes and poor health contributed to her obesity, and she argues that her obesity became a disease requiring surgical intervention.

> Bea: "Of course, it's a disease. A lot of people don't realize being overweight is a disease. And mine is caused by an underactive thyroid ... So that's how Medicare is paying for mine, because I have problems that caused me to become obese."

Bea also agrees with the ideal patient archetype's guidelines for an appropriate attitude. She believes that bariatric surgery requires patients to be vigilant about their health, and she describes surgery as "a tool for the rest of your life." Bea believes that bariatric surgery, as a surgical tool, actively teaches post-operative patients to take responsibility for monitoring their food intake: "Because if you eat sugar, even if it's a year from now, it can make you very, very sick." Bea willingly takes responsibility for post-surgical self-monitoring; in doing so, she is subscribing to the ideal patient attitude.

While Bea is quick to validate physiological and attitudinal aspects of the ideal patient archetype, she concurrently dismisses many ideal patient archetype aspects that deal with appropriate behavior guidelines. For instance, Bea failed to attend recommended support groups before or after her surgery. She also believes that pre-surgical psychological evaluations are worthless and poorly executed. Additionally, she was a long-time smoker, and only briefly gave up cigarettes before surgery, as was recommended by her surgeon. With all of these aspects, Bea asserts that there is a difference between being a good bariatric patient and following all of her surgeon's recommendations. For example, when discussing smoking, Bea states

> Bea: "I can't say that I will be smoke-free for the rest of my life, because it's not something I wanted to give up. I had to give it up. And there's a difference. Until I want to give it up, I will probably end up going back to smoking."

By casting morbid obesity as a disease that she wants to be rid of, and smoking as an activity that she does not want to give up, Bea is contesting surgical authority and guidelines for appropriate behavior. However, Bea does not define herself as a bad patient or a surgical failure. Bea truly believes that she is subscribing to all of the necessary and significant components of the ideal patient criteria. Bea recognizes the existence of other components, such as quitting smoking, undergoing psychological evaluations and attending support groups, but dismisses them as unnecessary.

Other mixed responders have similarly ambivalent reactions to the ideal patient criteria. Nicki, a 34-year-old stay-at-home mom, is extremely enthusiastic about the behavioral components of the ideal criteria. She calls her pre-operative patient orientation course "essential ... essential" and feels it is very important to participate in online support groups, calling them "So much knowledge!" At the same time that Nicki advocates for appropriate patient behavior, she also indicates disbelief in the inherent legitimacy of other criteria. For instance, Nicki does not draw upon the appropriate patient attitude when she claims that she had surgery because "I kind of like drastic things, drastic things work for me." She does not frame her surgery as a tool, nor does she talk about feeling personally responsible for successful weight loss. Nicki also shows ambivalence toward medical guidelines for physiological limitations.

> Nicki: "You just have to really meet the BMI standards. To tell you the truth, I had to gain a little weight to meet the standards for [my surgeon] because you have to be a 40. Or you have to have comorbidities and be over 35 – but I didn't have any. So I gained a little weight before I went to see him."

Nicki believes that strict BMI standards for patient selection are unnecessarily arbitrary. As Nicki knew that she did not meet the BMI standards, she altered her body to qualify for surgery. She feels no guilt or apprehension when she negatively conceptualizes physiological requirements as bureaucratic. However, Nicki does not dismiss all medical guidelines; she believes that it was very important to adhere to behavioral aspects of the ideal. Nicki, like Bea and other mixed responders, selectively chose to agree with some elements of the ideal archetype and discount other elements.

Like Nicki and Bea, mixed responders alternately embrace and reject ideal patient archetype components. They feel that some aspects are appropriate and valid, and other aspects are unrealistic or otherwise unimportant. The aspects of the ideal archetype that mixed responders choose to accept are frequently imbued with personal meaning. Just as Nicki feels it is important to adhere to behavioral components, and Bea strongly believes that her obesity surgery is a tool that will help her to eat better, all mixed responders indicate that some aspects of the ideal archetype have significant, positive meaning for them. By differentiating between appropriate and inappropriate criteria, mixed responders reject embracers' belief in limitless surgical authority. Mixed responders also reject embracers' frequent view that weight loss surgery is central in their lives. This ideological rejection of ideal patient components appears somewhat differently in strategizers' narratives.

Strategically Negotiating the Ideal

A few respondents were critical of the patient guidelines that comprise the ideal archetype. After encountering ideal patient components, three respondents felt that medical guidelines were generally worthless and unimportant. They understand archetype components as illegitimate gatekeeping devices limiting patients' access to surgery. Concurrently and seemingly contradictorily, they are also critical of the bariatric surgery industry's profit motive, and believe surgeons are more interested in making money than in enhancing patient care. These respondents did value their surgeries, however, and they explain how they *strategically* complied with ideal patient archetype guidelines. As strategizers, they intentionally acted appropriately in order to access weight loss surgery. However, unlike embracers or mixed responders, strategizers remain actively critical of the medical criteria they encounter. Strategizers indicate their negative views by critically complying with archetype components: they fulfilled physiological, diet, behavioral and attitudinal criteria, but are concurrently critical of these standardized medical guidelines. Strategizers recognize their nonconformity but do not see themselves as bad patients; rather, they view themselves as good patients who had been asked to jump through ridiculous hoops.

Criticism of the ideal archetype is apparent within strategizers' narratives. For instance, Fran, 53, indicates that patient guidelines are pointless. At Fran's first bariatric surgery appointment, she was asked to write down her dieting history for the surgeon's review. While Fran had recounted a decades-long dieting history in our interview ("I've gone through the Cambridge diet, Optifast, Dexatrim, exercise programs, walking, Vitamin B-12 shots, the Nutrisystem. You name it, I've done it."), she criticized the surgical group's request.

> Fran: "Who the hell keeps [diet history] records? Who has the time, you know? ... So, my husband and I, here we are making up these fake dates to try and make up a year [of a dieting history], and then the doctor picks it up, and discusses the year I 'dieted', and I'm thinking, 'What the hell?'"

Fran's objection to documenting her dieting history is rooted in her belief that she shouldn't have to grovel or recall former events in order to undergo surgery. Her attitude is distinctly different than embracers, who understand medical requests for information as legitimate. By creating a fictitious dieting history, Fran strategically manipulated the medical guideline requiring patients to have an appropriate, documented dieting history.

Throughout Fran's narrative she indicates privileging personal insights over medical regulations. For instance, Fran discounts her surgeon's recommendation that she understand support groups as integral to successful weight loss; however, in our interview she states that she might attend support groups if they were held at convenient times. Fran also understood psychological interventions differently. Rather than thinking about psychological testing as a one-time screening device, as her surgeon had framed it, she intends to undergo long-term therapeutic counseling in order to come to terms with multiple personal issues. With each ideal patient category, Fran indicates that her own insights and experiences trump medical advice. While Fran intentionally complied with medical criteria in order to access surgery, she does not embrace these guidelines.

Fran's strategic attitude toward surgery was similar to Iris's. Iris, 39, had undergone bariatric surgery a year before our interview and, while she was satisfied with her 76 pound weight loss and her surgeon's surgical performance, she indicated dissatisfaction with many non-surgical aspects of the bariatric industry. This frustration can be seen when Iris talks about how her mother (who also had bariatric surgery) was initially denied admittance into bariatric programs. Multiple surgeons had told Iris's mother that she was not obese enough to qualify for surgery.

> Iris: "My mom went to three different surgeons and one guy said, "Well you know, you don't look so bad." And I told my mom, "You should've asked if he'd sleep with you. And if he said 'No' ...""

In her interview, Iris suggests that surgeons' guidelines for permitting patients to access surgery are rooted in the medical field's subjective bias. Iris believes that physiological standards for surgery are set too high and are adhered to too stringently. Iris strongly feels that she is a better judge of her mother's surgical suitability than the surgeons. In contrast to her mother's rejection, Iris easily met physiological surgery qualifications, and eventually Iris's surgeon also operated on her mother. While she feels her surgeon's performance was satisfactory, Iris states that her surgeon was in business to make money. She claims, "It's just like a business. It's a well-oiled machine in his office." When Iris accompanied her mother on a post-surgical follow up appointment, the surgeon failed to remember that Iris was also his former patient: "He didn't even recognize me. It's such a business." She similarly believes that other surgeons are also motivated to have high patient loads and have high profits. As Iris's statements about surgeons indicate, she believes that weight loss surgeons are overly swayed by money and, concurrently, that surgeons have too much power in excluding patients from surgery. Though these sentiments are somewhat contradictory, they underscore her skeptical attitude and provide Iris with personal validation for approaching surgery strategically.

Iris, similar to other strategizers, is critical of the pre-surgical requirements her surgeon wanted her to follow. For instance, Iris indicates attending a pre-surgical orientation meeting strictly so that she could sign the attendance sheet and, thus, fulfill the mandatory meeting requirement.

She purposefully complied with behavioral components of the ideal archetype, including undergoing physiological and psychological examinations, so that she could undergo surgery. However, after having surgery, Iris thinks that she has done enough to satisfy her surgeon's requirements. She is unwilling to attend surgeon-sponsored support groups or speak about her experience at orientation seminars. She is also unwilling to keep post-surgical appointments with her surgeon.

Iris: "I'm not mad at him or anything. He did a good job. He did a great surgery. But to go for my four month follow up with him? I'm just not going to bother. I have all the care I need here. ... He's not doing any nutritional thing or anything, so why bother? It's not that I'm angry or anything, it's just it would be a waste of my time. So I'll call to cancel."

In this statement, Iris indicates that her post-surgical non-compliance is not related to her opinion about her surgeon's competence ("He did a good job.") or some personal dissatisfaction ("It's not that I'm angry or anything ..."), but rather that she does not recognize valid medical rationale for visiting her surgeon once her surgery was complete. Iris thus demonstrated her rejection of archetypical appropriate patient behaviors.

Like other strategizers, Iris believes that her weight loss success is linked to her personal choices rather than her ability to follow medical dictates. She feels that she knows how to handle her body after surgery. For instance, though Iris was told not to eat food and drink liquid at the same time (a common post-surgery behavioral recommendation), she says, "But I've stopped that. I don't wait a half-hour after eating to drink. I just can't. And my weight loss, it seems to be pretty progressive, and, so, I don't think it's injuring me." Here, Iris clearly views herself as a competent medical consumer and decision-maker.

Instead of viewing surgery as a tool or as a lifelong journey, strategizers primarily understand their surgeries as one-time medical procedures, like undergoing surgery for gallbladder removal or appendicitis. By understanding weight loss surgery strictly as a medical procedure, strategizers reject the ideal patient attitude. They do not believe that medically dictated forms of self-monitoring are crucial to their weight loss, though many strategizers indicate superficially complying with attitudinal expectations before undergoing surgery. This is seen, for instance, when strategizers attend mandated appointments and keep their true opinions silent. Also, strategizers frequently look down upon patients who strongly adhere to the ideal patient attitude. They critique patients who appear overly invested in their surgical identities, for example, those who carry around "before-and-after" photos or primarily socialize with other bariatric patients.

In sum, strategizers comprehend the significance of ideal patient archetype components and understand that it is necessary to comply with the archetype in order to access surgery. Strategizers distinctly assert that medical guidelines, though powerful, are often illegitimate and inappropriate. As is evident through this claim, strategizers have a different view of weight loss surgery than embracers, who value patient guidelines, or mixed responders who validate some of the criteria and dismiss others. While there is not a significant sample of strategizers, I did notice that strategizers, unlike embracers and mixed responders, did not portray obesity as a stigmatized identity within their narratives. This initial finding suggests that individuals' perception of obesity stigma as personally problematic may be linked to their negotiations of the ideal patient archetype.

CONCLUSIONS

This research demonstrates the significant role that medical guidelines play in shaping patients' health care experiences. All weight loss surgery patients are compelled to negotiate the terrain of bariatric surgery discourses in order to access surgery. All respondents encounter the ideal patient archetype as they prepare for surgery, and all engage in discourse negotiation. Some respondents embrace the ideal patient frame and validate all medical recommendations. Others, in contrast, are more critical of the ideal archetype. Mixed responders indicate balancing respect for medical authority with validation of their personal experiences. Strategizers validate their personal expertise and critically viewed medical guidelines as illegitimate. Regardless of each respondent's personal response to the ideal archetype, all respondents' personal narratives and health care experiences are influenced by their interactions with medical discourses.

An overwhelming number of research respondents embrace the ideal patient archetype and this finding should not be seen as generalizable to the broader population of weight loss surgery patients. The frequent presence of embracers may reflect the effectiveness of the ideal patient guidelines as selection procedures, as prospective patients who might have fit into the mixed responder or strategic categories may have been "weeded out" by surgeons. Additionally, research design likely impacted the types of respondents who participated, as participants were primarily recruited from an online message board/support group. Embracers may be the primarily users of this online site. Future research may look at weight loss surgery patients recruited from other sources.

This study reveals that the ideal patient archetype is a result, in part, of surgical controversies. Debates over surgical safety and its inherent value, as well as debates regarding surgical authority have created an environment where patient attributes are scrutinized. Surgical controversies have coalesced into a complex bariatric surgery discourse. The ideal patient archetype has become a central mechanism by which patients come into contact with bariatric discourses. That is, in the case of bariatric surgery, discourses become evident to patients through the employment of a discursive mechanism or frame. In this study, the frame I identify is the ideal patient archetype. Medical debates about bariatric surgery have impacted proponents' discursive conceptions of surgery. As I have demonstrated, the institutional logic of the bariatric surgery field corresponds with the ideal patient archetype. The resulting patient guidelines, which individuals are compelled to interact with in order to have surgery, make bariatric discourses tangible to patients. Institutional bariatric surgery debates can, thus, indirectly impact patients' health care experiences and conceptions of bariatric surgery. I have also found early evidence that patients' broader self conceptions may be notably impacted as they negotiate the ideal archetype. I will examine the impacts of bariatric discourse and ideal archetype negotiations on patients' self conceptions in future work.

When identifying the discursive frame that connects patients with medical discourses, I am also bringing discourse and framing studies into closer connection with narrative studies. Discursive frames can act as a mediating force between large social discourses and individuals' self-narratives. In recognizing the role discursive frames play in shaping patients' health care experiences, I build upon the work of interpretative practice scholars James Holstein and Jaber Gubrium (2000) by helping to clarify the process through which socially located individuals engage in social life.

Finally, this study reveals the continuing significance of medicalization. The bariatric field has harnessed historical and contemporary bariatric surgery debates and controversies in creating the ideal patient archetype, which directly influences patients' health care experiences. One outcome of the development of this discursive frame is that weight loss surgery is cast as an appropriate obesity solution when properly regulated. Additionally, individual patients are provided with a script to understand their surgical participation as medically valid, so long as they comply with the ideal patient guidelines. In future research it would be useful to explore if and how ideal patient guidelines influence public opinion of bariatric surgery as a medically appropriate obesity solution.

NOTES

1. This research project was reviewed and approved by the University of California, Santa Barbara's Human Subject Research and Review Committee.

2. The American Society for Bariatric Surgery (ASBS) formally changed its name to the American Society for Metabolic and Bariatric Surgery (ASMBS) in August 2007.

3. Definitions for "healthy weight," "overweight," "obese," etc. are constructed and occasionally contested within the medical community (see Saguy & Riley, 2005).

4. Three respondents regretted undergoing surgery. Of these, one respondent is classified as an embracer; she learned about the ideal archetype after her surgery and believes that her surgeon did not sufficiently implement it. The other two respondents who regret surgery indicated that they have mixed views of the ideal patient archetype.

ACKNOWLEDGMENT

I would like to thank Denise D. Bielby, Lisa Leitz, and Brooke Neely for their helpful comments.

REFERENCES

Altheide, D. (1996). *Qualitative media analysis.* Thousand Oaks, CA: Sage.

American College of Surgeons (ACS). *American college of surgeons bariatric surgery center network accreditation program manual.* (Retrieved March 27, 2007 (http://www.facs.org/cqi/bscn/program_manual.pdf)) Chicago, IL: American College of Surgeons.

American Society for Metabolic and Bariatric Surgery (ASMBS). (2007a). *Bariatric surgery fact sheet* (Retrieved June 1, 2007 (http://www.asbs.org/Newsite07/media/asbs_fs_surgery.pdf)). Gainesville, FL: American Society for Metabolic and Bariatric Surgery (ASMBS Press Kit).

American Society for Metabolic and Bariatric Surgery (ASMBS). (2007b). *American society for bariatric surgery fact sheet* (Retrieved June 1, 2007 (http://www.asbs.org/Newsite07/media/asbs_fs_asbs.pdf)). Gainesville, FL: American Society for Metabolic and Bariatric Surgery (ASMBS Press Kit).

Boero, N. (2007). All the news that's fat to print: The American "obesity epidemic" and the media. *Qualitative Sociology, 30,* 41–60.

Bordo, S. (1993). *Unbearable weight.* Berkeley: University of California Press.

Centers for Disease Control (CDC). (1999). Obesity epidemic increases dramatically in the Unites States: CDC director calls for national prevention effort. Division of Media Relations, October 26. Retrieved June 13, 2007 (http://www.cdc.gov/OD/OC/MEDIA/pressrel/r991026.htm).

Charmaz, K. (1994). Identity dilemmas of chronically ill men. *The Sociological Quarterly, 35*, 269–288.

Cheek, J. (2004). At the margins? Discourse analysis and qualitative research. *Qualitative Health Research, 14*, 1140–1150.

Collins, P. (2003). Storying self and others: The construction of narrative identity. *Journal of Language and Politics, 2*, 243–264.

Conrad, P., & Schneider, J. (1980). *Deviance and medicalization: From badness to sickness.* St. Louis: C.V. Mosby.

Encinosa, W., Bernard, D., Chen, C-C., & Steiner, C. (2006). Healthcare utilization and outcomes after bariatric surgery. *Medical Care, 44*, 706–712.

Evans, B. (2006). Gluttony or sloth: Critical geographies of bodies and morality in (anti)obesity policy. *Area, 38*(3), 259–267.

Everingham, C., Heading, G., & Linda, C. (2006). Couples' experiences of postnatal depression: A framing analysis of cultural identity, gender and communication. *Social Science and Medicine, 62*, 1745–1756.

Ferris, J. (2003). Parallel discourses and "Appropriate" bodies: Media constructions of anorexia and obesity in the contrasting cases of Tracey Gold and Carnie Wilson. *Journal of Communication Inquiry, 27*, 256–273.

Flum, D. R., Salem, L., Broeckel Elrod, J. A., Dellinger, E. P., Cheadle, A., & Chan, L. (2005). Early mortality among medicare beneficiaries undergoing bariatric surgical procedures. *Journal of the American Medical Association, 294*, 1903–1908.

Foucault, M. (1969). *The archeology of knowledge.* France: Editions Gallimard.

Gimlin, D. (2002). *Body work: Beauty and self image in American culture.* Berkeley: University of California Press.

Gimlin, D. (2007). Accounting for cosmetic surgery in the USA and Great Britain: A cross-cultural analysis of women's narratives. *Body and Society, 13*, 41–60.

Goffman, E. (1974). *Frame analysis.* Boston, MA: Northeastern University Press.

Goldberg, C. (1996). More people opting for surgery to treat obesity. *The New York Times,* December 31. Retrieved on May 15, 2007 (http://query.nytimes.com/gst/fullpage.html? res = 9B07E6DC1030F932A05751C1A960958260).

Grady, D. (2004). Operation for obesity leaves some in misery. *The New York Times,* May 4. Retrieved on May 15, 2005 (http://query.nytimes.com/gst/fullpage.html? res = 9B01E6D7133DF937A35756C0A9629C8B63).

Griffen, W., Bivins, B., & Bell, R. (1983). The decline and fall of the jejunoileal bypass. *Surgery, Gynecology, and Obstetrics, 157*, 301–308.

Guadagnino, C. (2007). Tracking bariatric surgery in New Jersey. *Physicians' News Digest,* June. Retrieved August 27, 2007 (http://www.physiciansnews.com/cover/607csnj.html).

Holstein, J. A., & Gubrium, J. (2000). *The self we live by: Narrative identity in a postmodern world.* New York: Oxford University Press.

Joanisse, L. (2005). "This is who I really am": Obese women's conceptions of the self following weight loss surgery. In: D. Pawluch, W. Shaffir & C. E. Miall (Eds), *Doing ethnography: Researching everyday life* (pp. 248–259). Toronto: CSPI/Women's Press.

Joranby, L., Pineda, K. F., & Gold, M. S. (2005). Addiction to food and brain reward systems. *Sexual Addiction and Compulsivity, 12*, 201–217.

Kushner, R. F. (2003). *Roadmaps for clinical practice: Case studies in disease prevention and health management – assessment and management of adult obesity: A primer for physicians.* Chicago, Illinois: American Medical Association.

Lawler, S. (2002). Narratives in social research. In: T. May (Ed.), *Qualitative research in action* (pp. 242–258). London: Sage.

Mason, J. (2002). Qualitative interviewing: Asking, listening, and interpreting. In: T. May (Ed.), *Qualitative research in action* (pp. 225–241). London: Sage.

Matthews Lovering, K. (1995). The bleeding body: Adolescents talk about menstruation. In: S. Wilkinson & C. Kitzinger (Eds), *Feminism and discourse* (pp. 10–31). London: Sage.

Monaghan, L. (2006). Weighty words: Expanding and embodying the accounts framework. *Social Theory and Health, 4*, 128–167.

National Institutes of Health (NIH). (1978). Surgical treatment of morbid obesity: Consensus Statement. National Institutes of Health Consensus Development Conference Statement. December 4–5. 1:39–41. National Institutes of Health, Washington, DC.

National Institutes of Health (NIH). (1991). Gastrointestinal surgery for severe obesity: Consensus statement. NIH Consensus Development Conference Consensus Statement. March 25–27. 9:1–22. National Institutes of Health, Washington, DC.

National Institutes of Health (NIH). (2004). *NIH releases research strategy to fight obesity epidemic* (August 24. Retrieved June 13, 2007 (http://www.nih.gov/news/pr/aug2004/niddk-24.htm)). Washington, DC: National Institutes of Health (NIH News).

Nestle, M. (2002). *Food politics: How the food industry influences nutrition and health.* Berkeley: University of California Press.

Oliver, E. (2006). *Fat politics: The real story behind America's obesity epidemic.* New York: Oxford University Press.

Rich, E., & Evans, J. (2005). "Fat Ethics": The obesity discourse and body politics. *Social Theory and Health, 3*, 341–358.

Riessman, C. K. (1983). Women and medicalization: A new perspective. *Social Policy, 14*, 3–18.

Saguy, A., & Riley, K. (2005). Weighing both sides: Morality, mortality, and framing contests over obesity. *Journal of Health Politics, Policy and Law, 30*, 869–921.

Salant, T., & Santry, H. (2006). Internet marketing of bariatric surgery: Contemporary trends in the medicalization of obesity. *Social Science and Medicine, 62*, 2445–2457.

Santry, H., Gillen, D., & Lauderdale, D. (2005). Trends in bariatric surgical procedures. *Journal of the American Medical Association, 294*, 1909–1917.

Shelton, N., & Johnson, S. (2006). "I Think motherhood for me was a bit like a double-edged sword": The narratives of older mothers. *Journal of Community and Applied Social Psychology, 16*, 316–330.

Silverman, D. (2000). Analyzing talk and text. In: N. Denzin & Y. Lincoln (Eds), *The handbook of qualitative research* (2nd ed., pp. 821–834). Newbury Park, CA: Sage Publications.

Stinson, K. (2001). *Women and dieting culture: Inside a commercial weight loss group.* New Jersey: Rutgers University Press.

Surgical Review Corporation (SRC). (2007). *Hospital based program: BSCOE requirements* (Retrieved May 20, 2007 (http://www.surgicalreview.org/pcoe/tertiary/tertiary.aspx)). Raleigh, NC: Surgical Review Corporation.

Thompson, D. (2001). Overweight and obesity threaten US health gains. *Surgeon General Press Release*, December 13. Washington, DC: US Department of Health and Human Services, Office of the Surgeon General. Retrieved October 11, 2005 (http://www.surgeongeneral.gov/news/pressreleases/pr_obesity.htm).

Throsby, K. (2006). Happy Re-birthday: Obesity surgery and the construction of identity. Paper presented at the "Surgical Solutions" seminar, May 6–7, 2006. McGill University, Montreal.

Throsby, K. (2007). "How could you let yourself get like that?": Stories of the origins of obesity in accounts of weight loss surgery. *Social Science and Medicine, 65*, 1561–1571.

United States Department of Health and Human Services (HHS). (2004). HHS Announces Revised Medicare Obesity Coverage Policy. *HHS News Release*, July 15. Washington, DC: United States Department of Health and Human Services. Retrieved June 13, 2007 (http://www.hhs.gov/news/press/2004pres/20040715.html).

Wann, M. (1998). *Fat! so? because you don't have to apologize for your size*. Berkeley, CA: Ten Speed Press.

Weber, M. (1949). "Objectivity" in social science and social policy. In: E. Shils & H. Finch (Eds & Trans.), *The methodology of the social sciences* (pp. 50–112). New York: Free Press.

World Health Organization (WHO), WHO Consultation on Obesity. (1999). *Obesity: Preventing and managing the global epidemic: Report of a WHO consultation*. Geneva, Switzerland: World Health Organization.

Zingmond, D., McGory, M. L., & Ko, C. Y. (2005). Hospitalization before and after gastric bypass surgery. *Journal of the American Medical Association, 294*, 1918–1924.

SECTION 3:
WOMEN AND SPECIALIZED HEALTH PROBLEMS

FROM THE PATIENT'S POINT OF VIEW: PRACTITIONER INTERACTION STYLES IN THE TREATMENT OF WOMEN WITH CHRONIC STDs

Adina Nack

ABSTRACT

Medical encounters are interactional/interpersonal processes taking place within contexts shaped by macro-level social structures. In the case of sexually transmitted diseases (STDs), medical encounters occur at a stigmatized crossroads of social control and gendered norms of sexual behavior. When women are diagnosed and treated for chronic STDs, practitioner demeanor has an important impact on how patients will view not only their health status but also their moral status. This chapter draws on in depth interviews with 40 women diagnosed with genital infections of herpes and/or human papillomavirus (HPV – the cause of genital warts) to explore three models of patient–practitioner interaction. The analysis focuses on the relationship between gender, construction of illness, and practitioner interaction style. In a broader context, the health risks posed by particular interaction styles to female STD patients shed light on

Care for Major Health Problems and Population Health Concerns:
Impacts on Patients, Providers and Policy
Research in the Sociology of Health Care, Volume 26, 95–122
Copyright © 2008 by Emerald Group Publishing Limited
All rights of reproduction in any form reserved
ISSN: 0275-4959/doi:10.1016/S0275-4959(08)26005-9

larger public health implications of combining morality with medicine for the broader range of patients with stigmatizing diagnoses.

Each year in the United States, millions of Americans become infected with one or more STDs (sexually transmitted diseases). I studied women living with HSV (herpes simplex virus) and/or HPV (human papillomavirus) infections because the long-term and unpredictable nature of these two chronic STDs typically result in serious illness experiences with negative ramifications for physical health, mental health, and interpersonal relationships. In addition, the incidence rates of both viruses are high, and, due to the fact that they are transmitted by skin-to-skin contact, their transmission rates are not necessarily decreased by the practice of "safer sex" techniques, such as the usage of latex male condoms. According to the Centers for Disease Control and Prevention (CDC, 2008a), "Nationwide, at least 45 million people ages 12 and older, or one out of five adolescents and adults, have had genital HSV infection ... Genital HSV-2 infection is more common in women (approximately one out of four women) than in men (almost one out of eight). This may be due to male-to-female transmission being more likely than female-to-male transmission." In terms of HPV, "Approximately 20 million Americans are currently infected with HPV, and another 6.2 million people become newly infected each year. At least 50% of sexually active men and women acquire genital HPV infection at some point in their lives" (CDC, 2008b).

My research focuses on women's experiences of being diagnosed with and treated for these STDs because the socio-historical constructions of sexual diseases (especially the gendered double-standard of sexual morality) have produced much stronger stigma for infected women than for infected men. While women's understandings of STD stigma do not begin at the diagnostic encounter (see Nack, 2002), practitioners play an important role in shaping the meanings that these patients attribute to their illnesses. This chapter presents the analysis of 40 female patients' experiences of interacting with medical practitioners during visits in which they received examinations, diagnoses and/or treatments for HSV and/or HPV. The analysis aims to expand medical sociological conceptions of practitioner interaction styles but to also begin to answer the question of how different practitioner interaction styles impact female STD patients' health outcomes (e.g., patient satisfaction, compliance, and overall well-being).

In this piece, I aim to answer the following questions. What practitioner–patient interaction styles do women with STDs experience? How can the example of women with STDs expand current medical sociological models of practitioner–patient interaction? What correlations exist between practitioners' sex/gender and interaction styles? What are the public health implications of different practitioner–patient interaction styles for the variety of patients with stigmatizing illnesses?

INTERSECTIONS OF MORALITY AND MEDICINE

The impact of social mores on health policies and social attitudes extends beyond sexual health. Several diagnoses continue to create "immoral patients," those who are judged according to the moral culpability of their conditions: for example, the mentally ill, alcoholics, drug addicts, smokers, and the obese. Gaussot's (1998) study of "good drinking" found that individuals either perceived alcoholism as a disease, a sign of creativity, or proof of social and moral failings. Smyth's (1998) sociohistorical analysis of female alcoholics found that social discourses portrayed alcoholic women as promiscuous, impoverished, and bad mothers. This gendered "moral outcast" model of female alcoholism promoted secrecy and denial amongst affected individuals.

Drug users have also employed denial as way to manage the stigma of being diagnosed as a drug addict. One study of injection drug users found that they were conflicted by internal contradictions: their saw themselves as responsible and careful injectors, but these self-concepts did not match their high-risk behaviors of lending and borrowing injecting paraphernalia (Plumridge & Chetwynd, 1998). The researchers determined that drug users resolved their identity contradictions via discourses of exoneration which fit the moral implications of the different risk behaviors. Sadly, the drug users put more energy into – and were more effective at – shielding themselves from moral stigma than at reducing high-risk behaviors.

Similarly, a lack of medical compliance has been found among individuals labeled by practitioners as obese. "If the fitness 'revolution' was driven by scientific findings about risk and behavior, it also took on a powerful moral and prescriptive dimension" (Brandt, 1997, p. 67). An interview study of obese patients found that each had been subjected to "contemptuous" treatment from their medical practitioners, and their resulting "fear[s] of humiliation prevents [them] from seeking health care" (Joanisse, 1999, p. 14).

SOCIO-HISTORICAL PERSPECTIVES ON STDs

By the late 20th century, epidemiological studies had shown behavioral choices to influence ill health. "No longer would disease be viewed as a random event; it would now be viewed as a failure of individual control, a lack of self-discipline, an intrinsic moral failing" (Brandt, 1997, p. 64). In contemporary society, many believe that illness is a consequence of individuals' poorly chosen, and hence irresponsible, behaviors. This mindset helps to explain why social prejudices intensify against individuals such as those infected with STDs who are believed to have caused their own stigmatization (Goffman, 1963).

The social histories of STDs in the United States and the United Kingdom reflect traditions not only of assigning responsibility to individuals with STDs, but also of differentially assigning stigma of moral character on the basis of sex/gender (Brandt, 1987; Davidson, 1994; Luker, 1998). Women with STDs, much more so than men, have been and continue to be socially constructed as morally culpable: they *earned* these diseases via promiscuous sexual behaviors that violated norms of feminine morality. Gendered social constructions of STD patients mirror the "double standard" in which "males are morally elevated by multiple sexual encounters while females are morally demeaned" (Eyre, Davis, & Peacock, 2001, p. 13).

The dominant ideology in our society has assigned stigma to certain kinds of patients (e.g., the obese, the sexually diseased, the mentally ill, the addicted), so how and why does the construction of stigmatized patients shape practitioners' interactions with such patients? Health care practitioners undergo professional training that is supposed to counteract underlying prejudice. However, research shows that practitioners are not always able to remain objective towards their patients: "In their encounters with patients, doctors may interpret personal problems and encourage individual behaviors in directions that are consistent with society's dominant ideological patterns" (Waitzkin, 1989, p. 225). As noted by Radley (1994), health care practitioners are not immune to stigmatized portrayals of disease: "How the doctor views the patient, whether the individual is seen to be a member of certain groups that are negatively stereotyped, can have an effect on how (or whether) treatment is carried out" (p. 103). For example, a recent UK study found that most male STD patients experienced relief from practitioner interactions that allowed them to voice their "sense of pollution experienced as disease" because the practitioners employed "strategic interactions" to protect patients' sexual selves (Pryce, 2001). In contrast, a study of HIV-positive women found that they experienced "stigma and discrimination" in interactions with medical practitioners: in general, female patients who are "assumed to be promiscuous may experience great difficulty in accessing appropriate medical care, support and services that are nonjudgmental" (Lawless, Kippax, & Crawford, 1996, p. 1373).

SEXUAL HEALTH INTERACTIONS: STIGMATIZED CROSSROADS

In addition to the control of health information and services, medical practitioners may serve the functions of being social control agents: they have implicit authority to attribute moral statuses to a variety of illnesses. Foucault (1978) asserted that social control has become more professionalized and oriented to the surveillance of deviant behavior. In particular, professionals' ability to intervene in and control others' behavior is enhanced by the discourse used by professionals to communicate specialized knowledge. His (1978) work on sexuality pertains directly to medical encounters. The ways in which both medical and lay people speak about particular diagnoses may denote blame and individual responsibility to the sick. Moral explanations for illness often serve the function of relieving public anxiety by defining illness as deserved punishment.

Scholars have asserted that sexuality has become medicalized and that one of the ramifications is the transformation of various aspects of sexuality into diseases: for example, homosexuality and fetishism (Foucault, 1978; Tiefer, 1996). This emphasis on medical aspects of sexuality resulted in a new morality of sexuality that has been cloaked in the legitimacy of science. Sexual "lifestyle" has become a key part of contemporary discourse on health and morality, such that medical research findings are used to support the moralization of sexual behaviors (Brandt, 1997; Luker, 1998).

This "science" of sexual morality is clearly evident in the moral agendas that have informed medical philosophy and public health services related to STDs. In 1909, the American moral reformer Mable MacCoy Irwin wrote, "I rejoice that they have put the scientific facts under our feet on which we may stand, as we tell our message of chastity to a sin-sick world" (as quoted in Luker, 1998, p. 613). Davidson (1994) argues that the ideology of the medical profession in the United Kingdom "viewed venereal diseases not just as a physical pathology but as the stigmata of the transgression of moral norms" (p. 271). During the period between World War I and World War II, he documents how "the moral surveillance and regeneration of patients came increasingly to be perceived as part of the functions of the VD treatment clinics in Scotland" (p. 272). In these eras of public concern about dreaded diseases, both reformers and practitioners "could call upon seemingly-neutral 'scientific' and medical information ... to argue to for a new moral, social, and sexual order" (Luker, 1998, p. 13).

Historically, public health campaigns and public opinion in both the United Kingdom and the United States have often targeted minority, sexually active, and working class women as the "vectors and vessels" of STDs (Davidson, 1994; Luker, 1998; Mahood, 1990). The social hygiene movement during the Progressive Era (1890–1913) was a time when medical practitioners and female moral reformers combine forces to more explicitly promote moral boundaries of sexual behavior in the pursuit of public health. However, these boundaries were gendered with regard to STDs: a doctrine of "physical necessity" justified men's forays into promiscuity. However, "the cowardly and cruel theory of innate depravity has been industriously disseminated as applying to 'fallen women' ... men the stronger, have remained free from blame; women the weaker have lived under a curse" (Dock, 1910, p. 60). For these reasons, I contend women's experiences of STD diagnostic and treatment interactions must be examined within the larger context of how female sexuality and sexual morality have been and continue to be constructed.

A modern merger of morality with medicine became evident when many Americans in the late 1980s displayed unsympathetic reactions to persons infected with HIV (Brandt, 1987). Eng and Butler (1997) argued that sexual mores are reflected in societal attitudes toward sexual health and, in turn, *explicitly* shape public health policy. Assigning moral culpability to illness may encourage policy makers to ignore environmental and social factors that contribute to disease and may reinforce the tendency to ridicule, reject or ignore those who suffer from a morally stigmatized illness. The intersection between science and sexual morality is further illustrated in the moral agendas that have informed medical philosophy and public health services related to other STDs. As contagious infections, genital HSV and HPV are the type of illnesses that represent "risks posed to the 'moral' by the 'immoral'" (Brandt, 1997, p. 71).

MODELS OF PRACTITIONER–PATIENT INTERACTION STYLES

Increased concerns for patient autonomy and interest in producing patient-centered outcomes have some bioethicists claiming that we are in an age of "new subjective medicine" in which "[p]atients' lives rather than patients' bodies will be the focus of medical interventions" (Sullivan, 2003, p. 1602). As such, the social roles of patient and practitioner are in flux. A survey of contemporary literature on physician–patient communication points to two general interaction styles: the "conventional *biomedical* approach [that] ignores the person with the disease" and the *patient-centered* model which "includes the conventional biomedical approach but that also goes beyond it to include consideration of the patient as a person" (Stewart, Brown, Weston, McWhinney, & Carol, 1995). These models fit well with two of the three patterns that emerged when coding my data on women's perceptions of their sexual health practitioners' interaction styles.

However, the literature does not provide a model that encompassed the third practitioner interaction style which emerged from my data analysis: I conceptualize this type as the *moral surveillance* model. In some ways, the foundation of this interaction style can be linked to early models of doctor–patient relationships that emphasized physician control (Ben-Sira, 1980; Friedson, 1970; Szasz & Hollender, 1956). However, this subset of practitioners, whom patients described as interacting via a moral surveillance model, exercised their authority in a manner that went beyond paternalism to communications of negative judgments about female patients' moral characters during medical encounters. In keeping with this conceptualization of the moral surveillance model, findings of a British cervical cancer prevention study can be read as evidence that this practitioner interaction style may be common beyond my sample: "In questioning women about their sexual history, doctors are using their authority to gain access to privileged information, and may be extracting a 'confession' without giving 'absolution'" (Posner & Vessey, 1988, p. 95). These researchers found that some doctors' subscribed to causal theories of how women contracted STDs which reflected negative beliefs about the women's characters: "The most frequently mentioned factor was 'promiscuity,' changing partners, or 'too much intercourse'" (Posner & Vessey, 1988, p. 91). As such, this practitioners were observed to have "offered a series of injunctions" during their interactions with their female STD patients (Posner & Vessey, 1988, p. 66).

THE IMPORTANCE OF STUDYING PATIENTS' PERCEPTIONS OF PRACTITIONER–PATIENT INTERACTIONS

Does the manner in which practitioners interact with patients to deliver health care have any significant impact on patients' health outcomes? Practitioner interaction style has emerged as an important determinant of patient satisfaction with both practitioner and medical treatment (Daly & Hulka, 1975; Korsch, Gozzi, & Francis, 1968; Spiro & Heidrich, 1983). "Patients rely heavily on the physician's mode of communicating when evaluating the care delivered by the physician" (Buller & Buller, 1987, p. 347). From the perspective of public health, this issue becomes more important because researchers have found that compliance may be largely a result of patient satisfaction (Korsch et al., 1968; Korsch & Negrete, 1972; Woolley, Kane, Hughes, & Wright, 1978).

In a study of the relationship between doctor–patient conversation styles and changes in health outcomes, researchers found that "more patient control (in the form of questions and interruptions) expressed during office visits was associated with improvements" (Kaplan, Greenfield, & Ware, 1989, p. 243). Anspach (1988) argues that the language used by medical staff and practitioners not only communicates information and organizes tasks but also reflects underlying attitudes and affects the delivery of patient care. Other research has found that, beyond verbal communication, "physicians' task behaviors carry socioemotional significance for patients" (Stewart & Roter, 1989, p. 194).

From a symbolic interactionist perspective, meaning is created interactionally, and communication strategies create, maintain, or transform social positions and roles. This chapter focuses on female patients interacting with practitioners during STD diagnoses and treatments, with the focus being on the women's perceptions of practitioners' interaction styles and the meanings created during medical encounters. The population in my study faced particular challenges in their medical encounters because their diagnoses represented incurable, contagious, and highly stigmatized conditions. Researchers studying non-stigmatizing yet chronic conditions found that doctor–patient interaction, whether perceived as positive or negative by patients, was highly significant in determining patient outcomes: "Doctors may in fact influence the outcomes of patients with chronic illness, not only by competent medical care, but also by shaping how patients feel about the disease, their sense of commitment to the treatment process, and their ability to control or contain its impact on their lives" (Kaplan et al., 1989, p. 244).

From a feminist public health perspective, I am primarily concerned with how practitioner–patient interactions impact patients who, by virtue of their gender, race, class, and/or age are usually in subordinate social positions. Even within medical encounters that do not involve sexual health, research has found that "patients (especially lower-income minority patients) may experience the powerful medical gaze of high-status professionals as morally judgmental as well as therapeutically curative ... their social disease is in the presence of medical surveillance" (Baker, Yoels, & Clair, 1996, p. 99). Friedson's (1970) critique of Parsons (1951) pointed out the importance of taking a conflict perspective on the asymmetry of physician–patient relationships: the mutuality of interest between patients and practitioners should not be overstated. Waitzkin (1991) describes the "therapeutic agenda" as the tendency for physicians to encounter patients with the narrow objectives of diagnosing and treating disease at the risk of ignoring the psychosocial aspects of patient care. However, he contends that class is the most important factor in physician–patient communication and ignores race and gender.

In this chapter, I investigate women's perceptions of interacting with the practitioners who diagnosed and treated them for chronic STDs: genital HSV and/or HPV infections. I seek to do more than merely describe and categorize interaction styles. I present a grounded theory (Glaser & Strauss, 1967) analysis of women patients' illness narratives and focus on their descriptions of communications with their practitioners. Via a grounded theory analytic approach and constant comparative analysis of the interview data (Glaser, 1978; Glaser & Strauss, 1967), three distinct types interaction style emerged from the data. In this chapter, I discuss the ways in which these models are similar to and differ from prevalent conceptualizations of doctor–patient interactions. I also explain how patients' experiences of different practitioner interaction styles shaped their self-conceptions of health and morality. Exploration of the ways in which female patients experience different practitioners' interaction styles provides insight to the nature and effects of practitioner–patient STD interactions. In addition, the findings of this study shed light on practitioner behaviors that may serve to increase or decrease the effectiveness of practitioner–patient communication in promoting positive patient health outcomes.

My goal is to uncover how professional norms of medical interaction, gender roles of both patient and practitioner, and stereotypes of sexual morality impact women's experiences of STD diagnostic and treatment interactions. First, I describe the research setting and methods. Next, I analyze the women's illness narratives to evaluate their perceptions of their practitioners' attitudes and behaviors. Then, I analyze the gendered nature of practitioner–patient STD interactions, looking at gender discrepancies in interaction style and in patients' preferences for practitioners on the basis of both gender and interaction style. Finally, I conclude by exploring how the women's diagnostic narratives illustrate broader implications of combining morality with medicine. Beyond STDs, these women's illness narratives point to micro-level effects of socially constructing patients as immoral (e.g., patients' satisfaction with medical interactions and overall well-being), as well as the macro-level public health implications of practitioner–patient interactions that may threaten patients' comprehension of and compliance with medical recommendations.

SETTING AND METHOD

Motivated by personal experience, I entered the setting as a "complete member" (Adler & Adler, 1987). At age 20, I had been diagnosed with a cervical HPV infection. Via self-education and involvement in STD education/outreach, I managed the stress of being diagnosed and treated. My investment in managing my sexual health status became the foundation for this research and provided me with the personal insights and clinical knowledge needed to connect with others facing STD diagnoses.

One of my concerns was practitioner–patient interactions. My goal was to understand patients' experiences of practitioner interactions; for this reason, their subjective perceptions became more important than any "objective reality." I realized that I was most interested in how practitioner interactions affected the patients and not in how the practitioners viewed themselves during these interactions as my focus of concern became the variety of factors that shaped female patients' experiences of STDs. While study of "the lived experience" carries its own set of limitations, I wanted to understand how the experience of the self and the body combine in an illness narrative. I decided to conduct an in-depth interview study of patients, focusing on female patients for this first part of the study. Literature on patient-centered medicine in family practice has found that patients' own ratings of care received are significantly strong measures of patient outcomes (Stewart et al., 1995). My goal was to analyze the women's accounts to discover what kinds of meaning they assigned to their interactions with practitioners, and, specifically, how they viewed the role of their practitioners in creating these meanings. This chapter focuses on my interview study of 40 women living with HPV and/or herpes who shared with me their experiences with sexual health practitioners during STD diagnostic and treatment encounters.

I constructed my research methods to reflect a reciprocal intention: before the women would give their stories to me, I would offer my support and resources as a sexual health educator. I also made it clear that, first as a volunteer and later as a professional sexual health educator, my assistance was available whether or not they chose to do an interview. However, I cannot be sure that very real power inequities of knowledge and expertise did not influence women's decisions to participate. The challenge was to locate myself as researcher in the "same critical plane as the overt subject matter" (Harding, 1987, p. 8). In this way, I viewed my values and actions as empirical knowledge that might either support or weaken my findings.

Obtaining approval from the university's committee on human research required that I not directly recruit subjects. Rather, subjects had to approach me, usually after hearing me present on sexual health, seeing my flyers in local clinics, or hearing about my research from other participants. Once interview subjects contacted me, I gained acceptance via my status as a sexual health educator and a complete member. At the completion of interviews, I would often ask participants to pass on my flyer if they knew another woman who might want to participate. In this way, I utilized snowball sampling to generate interviews (Biernacki & Waldorf, 1981).

Many researchers have criticized traditional methods of interviewing that emphasize distance, instead these researchers answer subject's questions, providing important educational information, and maintaining friendships with participants long after studies reach completion (Nielsen, 1990). During the interviews, I used researcher self-disclosure to create and maintain rapport, and I included self-reflexive reporting of the interview process as part of the transcribed data that I analyzed (Reinharz, 1990).

I conducted conversational, semi-structured interviews with consensual subjects who had all been diagnosed with genital herpes and/or HPV (including external genital warts and cervical lesions). Approximately 87% of the women lived in the Denver-Boulder metro area, with about 13% of my interviews being conducted by phone with women living in other states. Semi-structured or unstructured interviewing has been favored by many researchers because it "produces non-standardized information that allows researchers to make full use of differences among people" (Reinharz, 1990, p. 19). The subjects ranged in age from 19 to 56.

This chapter draws on the 40 women's descriptions of diagnostic and/or treatment interactions with 62 different practitioners: 40 female and 22 male sexual health practitioners. Some patients had been diagnosed with more than one STD; others had switched practitioners after receiving initial diagnoses. The interview gave each woman the opportunity to discuss with me her unfolding experiences with specific sexual health issues. I conducted the interviews in private locations of the subjects' preference. Informed consent forms assured all participants that pseudonyms would be used in all written research derived from this study. The interviews lasted from 45 minutes to 2 hours and were tape recorded with the permission of the subjects. When appropriate, I concluded the interview be reiterating offers of sexual health information and resources, either in the form of health education materials or referrals.

Methodologists have criticized single interviews for offering a glimpse into a life rather than the whole story. Given the sensitive subject matter (willingness to participate was dependent upon only having to be interviewed once) and transitory nature of the sample (approximately 75% graduate or undergraduate college students) made it improbable for me to incorporate follow-up interviews into the design. Inherent in the absence of follow-up interviews, was my inability to receive all participants' input on my final data analysis. Fortunately, I remained in contact with six participants after conducting their interviews. I asked for and received their input on preliminary drafts of chapters from this study.

I analyzed the data according to the principles of grounded theory (Charmaz, 1988; Glaser & Strauss, 1967), using constant comparative methods (Glaser, 1978) to adjust analytical categories to fit emerging theoretical concepts. Over time, I verified some categories and discarded others as data patterns reappeared. Initially, I sorted descriptions of practitioner interactions into levels of comfort/discomfort as recalled by the patients. Then, I re-examined the data with a focus on the particular aspects of each interaction that the patients causally attributed to their own emotional responses.

With each interview, I clustered subjects' experiences around particular levels of comfort/discomfort and causal attribution to assess the validity of my emerging three-tier model. The resulting evolutionary analysis was what Wiseman (1970) called a "total pattern," a sequence of events that held true for the overwhelming majority of those studied. I followed this plan of data collection and analysis to maximize the validity of my findings.

Analysis of patients' perceptions found that all 62 of the practitioner– patient interactions fit into one of the following exhaustive and mutually exclusive models of interaction style: the moral surveillance model, the biomedical model, and the patient-centered model. I coded each of the patient's descriptions of practitioner interaction to identify (1) the level of emotional distress or comfort that the patient attributed to a practitioner's interactions with her; and (2) the specific interactions described by the patient as having shaped her perceptions of that practitioner.

Interactions were coded as fitting the moral surveillance model if the patient described a high level of emotional distress resulting from the interaction and attributed this distress to specific instances of the practitioner demonstrating moral condemnation of her. To be coded as a moral surveillance interaction, the patient had to explicitly describe feelings of being judged as immoral by the practitioner. In contrast, I coded a patient's perception of a practitioner as fitting the biomedical model if the patient described a moderate level of emotional distress as a result of the practitioner interaction and attributed this distress to specific instances of the practitioner treating her in a reductionist manner (i.e., as a sick body part) and using words and/or actions that made her feel intimidated from asking questions. Finally, patients' perceptions of practitioner interactions were coded as fitting the patient-centered model if the patient described a low level of emotional distress and attributed her comfort to specific instances of the practitioner treating her as a whole person dealing with psychological and interpersonal ramifications as well as physical consequences. In addition, to be coded as a patient-centered interaction, the patient had to explicitly use positive adjectives in her description of the encounter (e.g., caring, nurturing, comforting). After conceptualizing these models and analyzing the data, I investigated the literature on doctor–patient interactions and compared my findings to others. Throughout this chapter, I incorporated relevant comparisons to demonstrate how my models confirm, expand upon, or differ from these existing models.

PRACTITIONER INTERACTION STYLES

All 40 women distinctly recalled how their practitioners presented their STD diagnoses and interacted with them during treatment encounters. The women's descriptions of 62 diagnostic and treatment encounters focused on all aspects of their practitioners' demeanor: what, how, and when the practitioners delivered the diagnoses. Their clarity and level of detail distinguished each practitioner and helped me to place them into one of these three categories of interaction style.

Moral Surveillance Model

The moral surveillance model surpasses Szasz and Hollender's (1956) most authoritative *activity-passivity* model in that the practitioner not only comes across as thoroughly dominant, but the patients also perceived this type of practitioner as condemning, and felt explicitly labeled as immoral during their STD diagnostic interactions. Practitioners who fit this interaction style exemplified Foucault's (1979) connection between knowledge and power in that these professionals exerted social control and were oriented toward the surveillance of deviant behavior. These practitioners behaved in ways that led their patients to view them as part of the medical elite who believed in the negative auxiliary traits of sexually diseased women: promiscuity, dirtiness, moral depravity, irresponsibility, and lack of intelligence. Of the patient–practitioner interactions described, 27% were coded as meeting the criteria of the moral surveillance model.

In some cases, the practitioners directly attacked the moral character and sexual conduct of their patients. Diana, a 45-year-old, single, African American professional remembered the accusations of her male gynecologist.

> At first I didn't know exactly what was wrong with me. I just knew that I was having some pain in my vagina. So I went to go see my gynecologist, and he said, "Well, you know, it looks like you had some really rough sex." Then, he actually asked, "Did you have some rough sex?" And I said, "Well, I didn't think it was rough – it was passionate." ... I thought I was going to die, literally die. And, I think that has probably been, up next to a doctor telling me I might need a transplant, probably one of the most devastating moments of my life – ever!

Many feminist scholars have documented the damaging social constructions of African-American women as a "Jezebel" character: hyper-sexual and "naturally" promiscuous, the kind of woman who would seek out "rough" sex (e.g., White, 1985). Diana's example illustrates how moral surveillance practitioners can be both sexist and racist.

In other cases, medical interactions left a patient feeling that her practitioner doubted both her level of virtue and her intelligence. These women felt as if they had been labeled morally inferior and incapable of avoiding sexual disease. Jasmine, a 20-year-old, White, upper-middle class undergraduate, described her encounter with a female practitioner.

> She's like, "Well, you've had unsafe sex?" And, I was like, "Yeah." She's like, "Well, you know the offer of free condoms here" ... And, I just wanted to pull out my SAT scores and be like, "Just look. I'm not stupid!" ... It really hurt because when you're trying to prove to yourself that you're a good person, and when you hear that from the

doctor it's very unsettling. And, you just walk off feeling like crap ... I remember crying and thinking how can I prove to her that this is not something that I normally do.

A third variation of the moral surveillance practitioner seemed to display general disgust and revulsion towards their patients. Chris, a 40-year-old, divorced, White professional recalled laying down with her feet propped up in gynecological stirrups that were hinged when her male gynecologist examined during her first genital herpes outbreak. "He just like looked at my crotch and said, 'Yep, that's herpes,' and sort of *slammed* my knees back together. He like smacked the sides of my legs...I felt shitty. Like, 'Let's close this back up.' You know, like a car, slam the hood down! Don't want to see anymore of this one." Treating the patient as the owner of diseased body parts illustrates an overlap between moral surveillance and biomedical model interaction style. However, only those practitioners who followed the moral surveillance model communicated negative perceptions of their patients' genital anatomy. Jasmine summed up the general complaint with moral surveillance practitioners: "Someone in the health field should be objective about it and should be there to help you and be there to answer questions and not be there to pretty much say, 'You've done the wrong thing.'"

Biomedical Model

The women viewed these practitioners as "aloof" and "matter of fact." Todd's (1989) study of communications between gynecologists and female patients found that while practitioners "concentrate on a biomedical approach to the body or organ," the patients' "biological concerns are embedded in broader contextual experiences" (p. 5). This type of practitioner embodies medical expertise by controlling communication flow and making all of the important decisions. Practicing medicine as neutral and scientific, these practitioners definitely sought the cooperation of their patients. However, the female patients' descriptions of diagnostic interactions reflected liberal use of the *medical gaze*, an interactional stance taught in medical schools that helps practitioners to remove their own and their patients' emotions from medical encounters (Baker et al., 1996). Of the patient–practitioner interactions described, 42% were coded as meeting the criteria of the biomedical model.

In some cases, the practitioners approached the work of medicine from a reductionist standpoint, considering the infected body parts as separate from a social and emotional human being. Summer, a 20-year-old, single, working-class Native American described her female gynecologist giving her a diagnosis of external HPV.

> She walks in like she's telling me I have a tonsil infection or something ... "Oh, you have genital warts." And I'm like, "Okay. So what's that? Are you gonna give me some pills?" And she explains to me that it's not curable. Then she gets me this mirror, and we're doing this funny little thing on the table and she's showing me what they look like. [*She didn't ask you if you wanted to see them?*]
>
> ... Well, I wanted to know, but it didn't feel very good because the moment I saw them, I knew that I'd seen them before, and I remembered who I had seen 'em on. Then she just walked out of the room and left me crying and thinking that I have this fucking disease that will never go away.

It was inappropriate for her practitioner to force her to view her infected genitalia. As illustrated, biomedical model practitioners may be oblivious to the emotional state of their patients, including the possibility that the women could feel both betrayed and angry with themselves for having trusted a partner with visible STD symptoms who had lied about the true cause of these symptoms.

Another variation of the biomedical model practitioner treated patients with blatant insensitivity, however not offering condemnation or explicit moral judgments. Sarah, a 24-year-old, single, Jewish graduate student's memory of her diagnostic interaction began with how her male gynecologist treated her during a cervical biopsy to check for HPV: "He left me with the parting message of: 'We'll find out if you have cervical cancer or not' ... I was contemplating infertility." Her practitioner was oblivious to the impact of his use of the word "cancer," and, in Sarah's case, this was enough to make her seek a female practitioner whom she hoped would show her more sensitivity. She recalled that this male physician was surprised that she was offended by his casual reference to the possibility of cancer.

However, seeking a female practitioner did not guarantee escaping the biomedical model interaction style. Rhonda, a 23-year-old, single, working-class Cuban American, recalled how her female gynecologist had delivered her diagnosis of genital herpes.

> It was very sterile throughout the entire experience. I went in, and she looked at me, and she said, "You have herpes." [*When you were still in the stirrups?*] Yeah, I think so; I think she just gave me a pamphlet. She didn't really tell me that much about it. But, she did tell me that I could not have unprotected sex because I could transmit it. And, I asked about oral sex, and she said, "No, because even when you don't have an outbreak, you can still transmit it." So, she made it seem like I could never receive oral sex again. And, I felt horrible!

Here, the practitioner's actions embodied efficiency and impersonality, leaving Rhonda feeling confused and too intimidated to ask for clarification. The women who had diagnostic and treatment interactions with biomedical model practitioners unanimously felt that the practitioners focused on treating the disease, not the patient.

Patient-Centered Model

When I concluded interviews by asking what advice these women would give to practitioners, all of them advised practitioners to be more holistic in regard to interaction style: e.g., "show more concern;" "make it easier to ask questions." In contrast to the two former types, the female patients perceived this third category of practitioners as compassionate and sensitive to the emotional implications of the diagnosis. This type of practitioner-interaction style has been well documented by Canadian researchers (Stewart et al., 1995): the patient's feelings are explicitly acknowledged by the practitioner, but the patient is not necessarily elevated to full participation. However, patient-centered practitioners do interact with their patients as human beings with agency who have multiple levels of concern (i.e., concerns beyond their immediate physical health and well-being). Of the patient–practitioner interactions described, 31% were coded as meeting the criteria of the patient-centered practitioner.

In all cases of this model, practitioners interacted with patients in ways that showed concern for non-physiological implications of STDs. Gita, a 23-year-old, single, middle-class Persian American described her diagnostic interaction with a female gynecologist.

> She didn't talk to me about HPV with my legs spread open. She put me in her office in a comfortable chair and talked to me. "How are you feeling? What's going on?" She really got deep with me – she took the time. She didn't just say, "We'll freeze them off, this is this, this is that, and you'll be fine." She explained that 70% of the population have it and how some people don't even know that they have it. She sat there with me and went over everything. And, then she said to me, "I give you permission not to look at your vagina for three weeks. I give you permission to feel okay because you're going to be okay."

Exemplifying a holistic stance, Gita's practitioner viewed her in her entirety – rational and irrational emotions included. This practitioner understood that simply telling a woman that her external warts were treatable was not enough to make her feel okay about seeing three-dimensional evidence of a contagious and possibly long-term disease on her genitalia.

In other cases, the practitioners put their patients at ease by taking extra time during both diagnostic and treatment interactions to anticipate questions and facilitate the patient getting all of her questions and concerns addressed. For Lily, a 40-year-old, widowed, White graduate student, the whole atmosphere of the clinic, in addition to her male gynecologist's interaction style, eased the diagnosis of a severe cervical HPV infection that would require a conization procedure (the most severe treatment before resorting to hysterectomy):

> He gained my confidence and was very respectful to me. They all treated me with an incredible amount of respect ... the nurses called you by your first name. It was warm, but there was also a lot of privacy ... I'm not afraid of asking questions, and, I made him explain everything to me ... Sometimes doctors don't like that, but this doctor preferred it. He preferred that I was involved in my own care and that I understood what was going on ... the doctor told me when I could expect to get the news. He called me himself, at home, and told me the results.

This practitioner's openness to his patient taking an assertive stance in asking questions, in addition to him taking the time to personally deliver her diagnosis distinguished him as a patient-centered practitioner. The majority of moral surveillance practitioners and biomedical model practitioner had less considerate ways of delivering diagnoses: ranging from not all (jumping straight into treatment without every sharing the diagnosis), to having staff leave messages on patients' answering machines (with no regard that the patient might share a phone line with family members or roommates).

Another variation of patient-centered practitioners displayed a more subtle empathy. Marissa, a 31-year-old, single, Hispanic graduate student explained how her male gynecologist put her at ease, both during the diagnosis and treatment for external genital warts.

> He was very nice because it was an awful thing. And I just felt lousy about the whole thing. So he just made small talk with me, but I felt so awful. [*He made you feel more okay about what was going on?*] Yeah. It was like this isn't a big deal. He just sat and talked to me about his daughter who played tennis and about my trip to London for the summer.

Marissa's practitioner recognized her distress, and gently distracted her so that her first wart removal was less traumatic. The women described patient-centered practitioners as coming to the STD encounter with assumptions that their patients may be experiencing both discomfort and shame. Patient-centered practitioners showed that they understood STDs as a social experience and interacted with patients in ways that were sensitive to the emotional and moral implications of their patients' diagnoses. This type of practitioner made sure to never give diagnoses when their patients were in compromising positions (e.g., half-undressed and legs up in stirrups).

Delivery of Healthcare Services

Both the practitioners' interaction style and also their gender affected patient interactions. Analysis of interaction style by gender reveals differences that are, in turn, reflected by female patients' preferences of not only particular interaction styles, but also practitioner's sex/gender. In addition, the women's illness narratives reveal several underlying health risks associated with practitioner interaction style.

Practitioner Sex/Gender: A Factor in Interaction Style

Parsons (1951) characterized patients as, "helpless, technically incompetent and too emotionally involved, therefore needing to put (themselves) into the hands of a professional who is technically expert, functionally specific and affectively neutral" (p. 456). Zola (1991) observed that this description of normative patient–doctor interaction roles sounded, "uncomfortably similar to the way in which society, through much of its history, has thought of female–male relationships" (p. 7). The data in this study support the relevance of gender roles and norms in how female patients view their interactions with sexual health practitioners.

Of the 62 sexual health encounters described, 40 were with female practitioners and 22 with male practitioners. Breaking down the frequency of practitioner interaction style by the gender of the practitioner revealed systematic patterns (see Table 1). A chi-square analysis was performed to determine the statistical significance of the association between practitioner gender and practitioner interaction style. Generally, male practitioners were overrepresented in moral surveillance interactions, and female practitioners were overrepresented in biomedical model interactions. The findings suggest that practitioner gender is an important and statistically significant factor in practitioner interaction style ($p < .05$). Slightly more than half of the female practitioners (52.5%) had been described as interacting in the biomedical model style, while the female patients had described half of the male practitioners (50%) as interacting through the moral surveillance model. More female practitioners (37.5%) than male practitioners (27.3%) were described as fitting the patient-centered model.

While sample size prevents any claims of generalizability, analysis of these data reveals intriguing questions and grounded theoretical explanations.

Table 1. Frequency of Practitioner Interaction Style by Sex of Practitioner $(n = 62)$.

Practitioner's Sex	Patient's Perception of Practitioner's Interaction Style			Total
	Moral surveillance model	Biomedical model	Patient-centered model	
Female	10%	52.5%	37.5%	64.5%
	(4)	(21)	(15)	(40)
Male	50%	22.7%	27.3%	35.5%
	(11)	(5)	(6)	(22)
Totals	24.2%	42%	33.8%	
	(15)	(26)	(21)	

$X^2 = 7.25, df = 2, p < .05.$

An alarming proportion of male practitioners fit the moral surveillance model of interaction. As the beginning of this chapter documents, research shows that the medical profession has long seen itself in the role of moral surveillance – especially on issues of sexual health. In keeping with Habermas' (1970) theory that science legitimates current patterns of domination, I propose that these factors combine with pervasive cultural constructions of females as inferior to foster misogynistic moralizing on the part of male doctors towards "fallen women."

Only 22.7% of the male practitioners were described as fitting the biomedical model of interaction style, but 52.5% of female practitioners fit this style. This gender discrepancy fits research findings on gender norms in many male professions, including medicine. Drawing on Hinze's (1999) study, the structure of the gender prestige hierarchy in medicine elevates masculine images and symbols. Therefore, I suggest that many female practitioners felt professional pressure and were socialized to *masculinize* their interaction style by employing interaction techniques such as affective neutrality, thereby pursuing a biomedical model approach with their patients. Acker's (1990) work supports this hypothesis, arguing that female professionals feel pressure to *de-emphasize* their feminine qualities in order to be successful in male hierarchical medical professions.

Even with the majority of female practitioners fitting the biomedical model, the majority of the female patients (82.5%) ultimately choose to see a female practitioner for sexual health services. Their choices may be evidence of the women's intuitive knowledge of gender disparity in moral surveillance interaction style. Approximately 38% of the women switched from seeing male practitioners for their first gynecological exams to seeing female practitioners for STD diagnosis and/or treatment. Gloria, a 48-year-old, single, Chicana graduate student explained her rationale for choosing female practitioners.

> I started demanding female doctors – I don't see male doctors anymore. I don't allow them to poke in my privates anymore ... They were insensitive, harsh with the way they would look in my area. I just didn't feel like they were gentle at all. Their hands were too big ... and it just didn't feel like they cared that much. That's what it was – I felt like cattle being herded through an office.

This strong preference reflects the women's fairly uniform rationale that female practitioners are more likely to interact with them in a patient-centered manner, which they often saw equivalent to exhibiting feminine traits (e.g., being good listeners, showing compassion, etc.). However, the female patients' overall views of female practitioners did not match their detailed descriptions of specific interactions with these same practitioners: 62.5% of the female practitioners fit either the moral surveillance or biomedical models of interaction style.

A minority of the women, 17.5%, switched to or continued to see male sexual health practitioners. Rhonda, a 23-year-old, single Cuban American explained her preference for male gynecologists.

> Women might be a little harder on you – they know where you're coming from, so they don't treat you with kid gloves. I think maybe a male doctor would treat you a little bit more cautiously because he's not really sure if he's treading on sensitive feelings. You know, he doesn't have firsthand knowledge of what you're going through and what's going on with you ... I think he might be more cautious.

Her rationale reflects the belief of a few women that a gender mismatch between patient and practitioner might lead to more polite interactions. In addition, I suggest that the small number of female patients who prefer and remain loyal to male practitioners might do so because of exposure to and belief in occupational gender norms of male prestige and expertise in medicine. However, as Pam, a 42-year-old White working-class graduate student pointed out, "class is an important factor in being able to choose a doctor by gender." She sees the fact that she ultimately was treated by a male practitioner as a result of socioeconomic restrictions that prevented her from being able to see a female practitioner, her true preference.

Interaction Style as Risk to Patient Health
Behind the statistics in Table 1 are stories about the health damage done to these female patients by practitioners who employed moral surveillance and biomedical model styles of interaction in the examination room.

The women's narratives revealed that practitioners who fit the moral surveillance and biomedical models of interaction style directly damaged patients' physical health because they were the most prone to delivering inaccurate and incomplete information. Moral surveillance and biomedical model practitioners were not empathetic and, therefore, failed to accurately predict what types of information their patients most needed during STD diagnostic and/or treatment encounters.

The data revealed that practitioners whose interaction styles could be classified under the moral surveillance or biomedical models were responsible for *every* case of a practitioner giving significantly incorrect medical information. Helena, a 31-year-old Greek-American graduate student, describes having been given incorrect and incomplete information about HPV. "There was never any discussion about [HPV] ... There was really no, 'this is what you should do, this is what you shouldn't do from now on' ... There wasn't any discussion like, 'And, you have this for the rest of your life, and you may get cervical cancer from it.'"

As illustrated by Helena's recollection, some of the biomedical model practitioners did not fully explain the chronic nature of herpes and HPV. The women in these situations reflected that while the absence of this vital information made them calmer in the doctor's office, they were more upset and confused later when they found out the truth from other sources (e.g., the internet, pamphlets, friends, etc.). Francine remembered feeling calm when she and her partner were given genital warts diagnoses, "because as far as we knew, once we got rid of them we didn't have this anymore." Similarly, Helena felt like her practitioner was going to treat her external genital warts, "and then everything was going to be fine ... because nothing else was really explained."

In addition, those practitioners who employed a moral surveillance style of interaction ended up damaging their patients' psychological perceptions of well-being. Diana remembered holding back her tears until after her practitioner had finished delivering her herpes diagnosis over the phone.

> I let down right after he hung up. I was crying all over the house. I was just a basket case then. I called my shrink and was just hysterical over the phone ... He said, "Well, I think you need to come in tomorrow, and we'll talk about it ... I was just devastated – I was very depressed. I remember getting in the bed, you know, just pulling the covers over my head and not wanting to ever come out.

Helena also left her diagnosis emotionally distraught: "I just came home from the doctor and felt so dirty." Jamie, an 18-year-old, White, upper middle-class undergraduate painfully recalled that she left her diagnostic interactions feeling, "like a slut," viewing her practitioner's moralistic attitude as a harbinger of the social ridicule to come.

In contrast to the above scenarios, one patient-centered practitioner turned the diagnosis and treatment for genital herpes into a positive medical encounter and an opportunity to assess the patient's total sexual health. Elle, a 32-year-old white, working-class graduate student, described her female practitioner as having used her diagnostic encounter to make her herpes diagnosis feel more manageable. The practitioner explained to Elle that, while herpes may be incurable, it also may not be forever a symptomatic condition. In addition, Elle's practitioner asked if she wanted to be tested for other STDs. Elle explained that being treated with respect helped her to respect the practitioner's recommendation, and she decided to get the "full screening" for STDs at that appointment.

CONCLUSIONS

The women's illness narratives portray sexual health practitioners most often as agents of health (biomedical model) and social control (moral surveillance model). However, they clearly express a preference for and appreciation of health agents with a holistic focus (patient-centered model). With regard to practitioner sex/gender, the women's preferences for female sexual health practitioners reflect an experiential desire to avoid practitioners who utilize a moral surveillance interaction style. Despite the fact that the women's accounts described only 37.5% of female practitioners as fitting the patient-centered model of interaction style, their overall selection of female practitioners coexists with an expressed preference for more patient-centered interactions. This contradiction of realities suggests that gendered expectations of feminine traits (ones that overlap strongly with patient-centered/holistic traits) may bias female patients' assumptions of female practitioners' interaction styles, thereby affecting their choice of female sexual health practitioners. Further research with a larger sample could help to illuminate the complex relationships between the sex/gender of both patients' and practitioners', practitioner interaction style, patient satisfaction/comfort, perceived interactional constructions of morality, and patient compliance.

There are public health costs of moral surveillance and biomedical interaction styles. First, this study and others have demonstrated that non-compliance with medical practitioners' recommendations for treatment and/ or behavioral changes is more likely to occur when a patients feel judged by their practitioners. Second, patients are less likely to feel comfortable asking questions and getting clarifications about diagnoses or treatment plans when they perceive their practitioners as being judgmental (moral surveillance model) or distant (biomedical model). This can lead to patients not understanding the nature (chronic or curable) or their illness or the ramifications of their illness for others (e.g., modes of transmission). Finally, an interaction with a practitioner who communicates condemnation of a patient based on that patient's illness can lead to that patient experiencing mental health trauma: for example, anxiety about how others will perceive them or depression over seeing themselves as a bad person who brought this illness upon themselves.

In contrast, there are public health benefits of more practitioners embracing a patient-centered interaction style. The patient-centered model of interaction can produce patients who will be more likely to follow medical treatment plans and modify risky behaviors because they will not only *understand* their medical pathways toward healing, but they will also *believe* that they deserve to get well. If promoting health is our goal, then we must protect the moral identities of patients and empower them to get the information they need during interactions with their practitioners.

In practical terms, how might we accomplish this goal? By changing the way we train health practitioners and by adding professional health educators to the medical team. This study shows how practitioner interaction style might introduce stigma and shame into patients' medical encounters. If public health is our goal, then we must train medical practitioners to interact with patients in ways which protect patients' views of themselves as "good" people who do not deserve their illnesses. Ideally, the style and focus of medical training would incorporate holistic goals of patient-centered healthcare. Realistically, professional and economic constraints make it likely for the biomedical model of practitioner interaction style to remain dominant. In this case, professional health educators should be added to the medical team. They can educate patients about symptoms and treatment options and also offer psychological/emotional support, complementary to the technical expertise provided by medical practitioners. Research on changing student physicians' views on authority in physician-patient relationships shows that "humanistic training" is partly responsible for a shift away from the biomedical model of interaction (Lavin, Haug, Belgrave, & Breslau, 1987). In the case of the moral surveillance model, I contend that there are public health benefits, in the form of patients' emotional well-being and compliance, to eliminating professional and social acceptance of this practitioner–patient interaction style. My study echoes findings of research on HIV treatment and counseling: safeguarding the moral statuses of patients is vital to achieving compliance (Plumridge & Chetwynd, 1998).

If we are to create effective treatment programs for stigmatized illnesses, then we have to eliminate the moral judgments of medical practitioners and the social constructions of these conditions being "deserved" and caused by "bad" behavior. Brandt (1997, p. 68) warned that unhealthy behaviors "such as cigarette smoking are sociocultural phenomena, not merely individual or necessarily rational choices." Therefore, labeling a health condition as deviant will not discourage individuals from engaging in high-risk and/or unhealthy behaviors. In the case of contagious illnesses, such as STDs, patient non-compliance can result in others becoming infected. While in the case of non-contagious illnesses, non-compliance may result in stress for caretakers or endanger the general public (e.g., driving under the influence of drugs or alcohol).

A concerted effort to promote the patient-centered model of practitioner–patient interaction can increase the numbers of patients who are compliant (with treatment plans and behavior modifications) because they will better understand the medical pathways toward healing *and* they will believe that they deserve to get well.

ACKNOWLEDGMENT

This chapter expands on ideas and research which appeared in my book, *Damaged Goods? Women Living with Incurable STDs*, ©2008 by Temple University Press.

REFERENCES

Acker, J. (1990). Hierarchies, jobs, bodies: A theory of gendered organizations. *Gender and Society, 4*(2), 139–158.

Adler, P. A., & Adler, P. (1987). *Membership roles in field research*. Newbury Park, CA: Sage.

Anspach, R. R. (1988). Notes on the sociology of medical discourse: The language of case presentation. *Journal of Health and Social Behavior, 29*(4), 357–375.

Baker, P. S., Yoels, W. C., & Clair, J. M. (1996). Emotional expression during medical encounters: Social disease and the medical gaze. In: V. James & G. Jonathon (Eds), *Health and the sociology of emotions*. Oxford: Blackwell Publishers.

Ben-Sira, Z. (1980). Affective and instrumental components in the physician–patient relationship: An additional dimension of interaction theory. *Journal of Health and Social Behavior, 21*, 170–180.

Biernacki, P., & Waldorf, D. (1981). Snowball sampling. *Sociological Research Methods, 10*, 141–163.

Brandt, A. M. (1987). *No magic bullet: A social history of venereal disease in the United States since 1880*. New York: Oxford University Press.

Brandt, A. M. (1997). Behavior, disease, and health in the twentieth century United States: The moral valence of individual risk. In: A. Brandt & P. Rozin (Eds), *Morality and health*. New York: Routledge.

Buller, M. K., & Buller, D. B. (1987). Physician's communication style and patient satisfaction. *Journal of Health and Social Behavior, 13*, 347–359.

Centers for Disease Control and Prevention (CDC). (2008a). Genital HPV infection – CDC fact sheet, March 5, 2008. Accessed online March 26, 2008 (http://www.cdc.gov/std/HPV/STDFact-HPV.htm).

Centers for Disease Control and Prevention (CDC). (2008b). Genital Herpes – CDC Fact Sheet January 4, 2008. Accessed online March 26, 2008 (http://www.cdc.gov/std/Herpes/STDFact-Herpes.htm).

Charmaz, K. (1988). The grounded theory method: An explication and interpretation. In: R. Emerson (Ed.), *Contemporary field research: A collection of readings*. Prospect Heights, IL: Waveland Press.

Daly, M. B., & Hulka, B. S. (1975). Talking with the doctor. *Journal of Communication, 25*(2), 148–152.

Davidson, R. (1994). Venereal disease, sexual morality, and public health in interwar Scotland. *Journal of the History of Sexuality, 5*(2), 267–294.

Dock, L. (1910). *Hygiene and morality: A manual for nurses and others, giving an outline of the medical, social and legal aspects of the venereal diseases*. New York: G.P. Putnam's Sons.

Eng, T., & Butler, W. (1997). *The hidden epidemic: Confronting sexually transmitted diseases*. Washington, DC: National Academy Press.

Eyre, S. L., Davis, E. W., & Peacock, B. (2001). Moral argumentation in adolescents' commentaries about sex. *Culture, Health and Sexuality, 3*(1), 1–17.

Foucault, M. (1978). *The history of sexuality, volume 1*. New York: Pantheon.

Foucault, M. (1979). *Discipline and power*. New York: Vantage.

Friedson, E. (1970). *Professional dominance*. New York: Atherton.

Gaussot, L. (1998). Representations of alcoholism & the social construction of "Good Drinking". *Sciences Sociales et Sante, 16*(1), 5–42.

Glaser, B. G. (1978). *Theoretical sensitivity*. Mill Valley, CA: Sociological Press.

Glaser, B. G., & Strauss, A. L. (1967). *The discovery of grounded theory: Strategies for qualitative research*. Chicago: Aldine.

Goffman, E. (1963). *Stigma: Notes on the management of spoiled identity*. Englewood Cliffs, NJ: Prentice Hall.

Habermas, J. (1970). *"Technology and Science as 'Ideology,'" from his toward a rational society*. Boston: Beacon.

Harding, S. (1987). *Feminism and methodology*. Bloomington: Indiana University Press.

Hinze, S. W. (1999). Gender and the body of medicine or at least some body parts: (Re)Constructing the prestige hierarchy of medical specialties. *The Sociological Quarterly, 40*(2), 217–239.

Joanisse, L. (1999). Fat bias in the delivery of health care. *Annual Meeting of the American Sociological Association*, Chicago, IL.

Kaplan, S. H., Greenfield, S., & Ware, J. E. (1989). Impact of the doctor–patient relationship on the outcomes of chronic disease. In: M. Stewart & D. Roter (Eds), *Communicating with medical patients* (pp. 228–245). Newbury Park, CA: Sage Publications.

Korsch, B. M., Gozzi, E. K., & Francis, V. F. (1968). Gaps in doctor–patient communication. *Pediatrics, 42*, 855–870.

Korsch, B. M., & Negrete, V. F. (1972). Doctor–patient communication. *Scientific American, 227*, 66–74.

Lavin, B., Haug, M., Belgrave, L. L., & Breslau, N. (1987). Change in student physicians' views on authority relationships with patients. *Journal of Health and Social Behavior, 28*(3), 258–272.

Lawless, S., Kippax, S., & Crawford, J. (1996). Dirty, diseased and undeserving: The positioning of HIV positive women. *Social Science and Medicine, 43*(9), 1371–1377.

Luker, K. (1998). Sex, social hygeine, and the state: The double-edged sword of social reform. *Theory and Society, 27*(5, October), 601–634.

Mahood, L. (1990). The Magdalene's friend: Prostitution and social control in glasgow, 1869–1890. *Women's Studies International Forum, 13*(1/2), 49–61.

Nack, A. (2002). Bad girls and fallen women: Chronic STD diagnoses as gateways to tribal stigma. *Symbolic Interaction, 25*(4), 463–485.

Nielsen, J. M. (1990). *Feminist research methods*. Boulder: Westview.

Parsons, T. (1951). *The social system*. New York: Free Press.

Plumridge, E. W., & Chetwynd, S. J. (1998). The moral universe of injecting drug users in the era of AIDS: Sharing injecting equipment and the protection of moral standing. *AIDS Care, 10*(6), 723–733.

Posner, T., & Vessey, M. P. (1988). *Prevention of cervical cancer: The patient's view*. London: King Edwards Hospital Fund for London.

Pryce, A. (2001). "The first thing I did when I came back from the clinic last week was change the sheets on the bed": Contamination, penetration and resistance – male clients in the VD clinic. *Current Sociology, 49*(3, May), 55–78.

Radley, A. (1994). *The social psychology of health and disease*. London: Sage.

Reinharz, S. (1990). *Feminist methods in social research*. Oxford: Oxford University Press.

Smyth, D. M. (1998). Common sense understanding of the female alcoholic, *Annual meeting of the society for the study of social sroblems*, San Francisco, CA.

Spiro, D., & Heidrich, F. (1983). Lay understanding of medical terminology. *The Journal of Family Practice, 17*, 277–279.

Stewart, M., Brown, J. B., Weston, W. W., McWhinney, I. R., & Carol, L. (1995). *Patient-centered medicine: Transforming the clinical approach*. Thousand Oaks, CA: Sage Publications.

Stewart, M., & Roter, D. (Eds). (1989). *Communicating with medical patients*. Newbury Park, CA: Sage Publications.

Sullivan, M. (2003). The new subjective medicine: Taking the patient's point of view on health care and health. *Social Science and Medicine, 56*(7), 1595–1604.

Szasz, T., & Hollender, M. (1956). A contribution to the philosophy of medicine: The basic models of the doctor-patient relationship. *AMA Archives of Internal Medicine, 97*, 585–592.

Tiefer, L. (1996). The medicalization of sexuality: Conceptual, normative, and professional issues. *Annual Review of Sex Research, 7*, 252–282.

Todd, A. D. (1989). *Intimate adversaries: Cultural conflict between doctors and women patients.* Philadelphia, PA: University of Pennsylvania Press.

Waitzkin, H. (1989). A critical theory of medical discourse: Ideology, social control, and the processing of social context in medical encounters. *Journal of Health and Social Behavior, 30*(June), 220–239.

Waitzkin, H. (1991). *The politics of medical encounters: How patients and doctors deal with social problems.* New Haven, Connecticut: Yale University Press.

White, D. G. (1985). *Ain't I a woman: Female slaves in the plantation south.* New York City, NY: W.W. Norton & Company, Inc.

Wiseman, J. P. (1970). *Stations of the lost.* Chicago: University of Chicago Press.

Woolley, F. R., Kane, R. L., Hughes, C. C., & Wright, D. D. (1978). The effects of doctor–patient communication on satisfaction and outcome of care. *Social Science and Medicine, 12,* 123–128.

Zola, I. K. (1991). Bringing our bodies and ourselves back. In: Reflections on a past, present, and future "Medical Sociology," *Journal of Health and Social Behavior, 32*(1), 1–16.

"I'M STILL HERE": A 10 YEAR FOLLOW-UP OF WOMEN'S EXPERIENCES LIVING WITH HIV

Donna B. Barnes

ABSTRACT

Women with HIV have increased longevity and the potential for decreasing mother to child transmission with the use of antiretroviral therapy. Since the beginning of the AIDS epidemic in 1980, the disease has evolved from an acute condition to a chronic one. How have women long-term survivors transitioned from a "death sentence" to living with HIV/AIDS as a chronic illness? In this study, we investigate the reproductive, mothering, and living experiences of HIV positive women 10 years after their participation in a study of their reproductive decisions. The sample was taken from two groups of women living with HIV ($n = 60$), one in Oakland, California ($n = 30$) and one in Rochester, New York ($n = 30$). Both groups participated in the initial study (1995–2001). The inclusion criteria for this study are women with HIV who are living and well enough to participate in a face-to-face interview. Of the original 60 women, 52 women are living. Two and one half years into this 4-year study, the author has completed interviews with 25 women from Oakland ($n = 10$) and Rochester ($n = 15$). An unexpected life with HIV challenges participants to live a viable life different from their

Care for Major Health Problems and Population Health Concerns:
 Impacts on Patients, Providers and Policy
Research in the Sociology of Health Care, Volume 26, 123–138
Copyright © 2008 by Emerald Group Publishing Limited
All rights of reproduction in any form reserved
ISSN: 0275-4959/doi:10.1016/S0275-4959(08)26006-0

pre-diagnosed life. It involves a life of defining normalcy in everyday experiences and building a legacy of a life worth living. Participants' issues and concerns of living with HIV/AIDS identify what kinds of cultural notions, and medical and social interventions support or undermine women's reproductive, mothering, and long-term living with HIV/AIDS.

INTRODUCTION

In 1996 highly active antiretroviral therapy (HAART) became available, decreasing mortality for people with HIV/AIDS. Since the beginning of the AIDS epidemic in 1980, the disease has evolved from an acute condition to a chronic one. Women with HIV thus have increased longevity and the potential for decreasing mother to child transmission (MTCT) with the use of antiretroviral therapy (ART) (Cohan, 2003; Connor et al., 1994). How have women long-term survivors transitioned from a "death sentence" to living with HIV/AIDS as a chronic illness? In this follow-up study we investigated the reproductive, mothering, and living experiences of HIV positive women 10 years after their participation in a study of their reproductive decisions.

The genesis for this study was the federally funded research project entitled "HIV-infected Women's Reproduction Decision Making Processes." Women's decisions were based on their judgment of the relative weight of positive aspects of motherhood versus the negative pressures of social and public opinion. Counteracting the often strongly negative message in their social environment were participants' personal views in favor of motherhood, which were present in varying combinations and degrees: their belief that motherhood offered them a reason to look to the future; a socially valued identity, particularly for participants with few other options for social approval; a chance to regain missed mothering experiences, often related to drug use; and their beliefs that God or a spiritual force was the ultimate authority, protector, and comforter.

The study's findings demonstrated that motherhood was dynamically centered in a participant's life course. This took place in a changing social and medical landscape, situating participants within an environment of the unpredictable likelihood of support and rejection from a variety of social relationships, and agencies, and uncertainties about their odds of living longer and having an opportunity to mother (Barnes & Murphy, 2009).

In this follow-up study, participants' mothering experiences were examined, along with what relationships supported or undermined the reproduction and mothering for these HIV positive women. What has it been like living long term with HIV? What are the issues for women living with HIV who have chosen not to have children as well as for women who had children prior to or while seropositive, given that women are living longer with the potential for improved medical care? What are their experiences of being a mother? Is there cultural support for mothers with HIV and where does it come from? Are women's personal beliefs about God supported by family, community, and religious groups? A unifying theme running through these questions is the importance of understanding the meanings women make of their lives and the socio-cultural contexts of interactions (Collins, 1994). Understanding HIV positive women's reproductive choices, mothering and lived experiences, particularly for long-time survivors, is imperative in order to address issues of medical treatment and social services.

BACKGROUND

In 1995 when this research on HIV positive women's reproductive decision making began, pregnant women with HIV/AIDS had few options. Providers' counsel, women reported, was most likely to advise termination of their pregnancies (Levine & Dubler, 1990). This advice was supported by the federal recommendation for prevention of transmission of HIV from mother to child. The official statement from the Centers for Disease Control and Prevention was that "Infected women (with HIV) should be advised to consider delaying pregnancy until more is known about perinatal transmission of the virus" (Centers for Disease Control and Prevention, 1985, p. 725).

During the 1980s and early 1990s, women were diagnosed later in the course of their disease and died sooner after their diagnoses than men (Sterling et al., 1999). Activists at the AIDS Conference in San Francisco in 1990 chanted, "AIDS is a disaster, women die faster" (Personal conversation, 2008). It wasn't until 1993 that the Centers for Disease Control and Prevention changed the definition of AIDS to a gender-neutral one based on CD_4 counts as well as incorporating opportunistic conditions/diseases that afflicted women (Centers for Disease Control and Prevention, 1993). Due both to earlier recognition of women's HIV status and also to the introduction of ART, women began to live longer.

Looking back over the last decade of medical advances and clinical interventions for women with HIV/AIDS, one of the most successful treatments has been the use of zidovudine to reduce MTCT (Connor et al., 1994). As more medications were discovered and combinations of medications tested, MTCT treatment became more available (Cohan, 2003). Women were encouraged to access prenatal care and to participate in ART therapy, which decreased MTCT dramatically (Fleming et al., 2002). This discovery brought about new medical concerns. If women were treated to reduce MTCT with ART while pregnant, it added to a woman's burden of life long use of particular kinds of ART and other drug combination therapies due to possible drug resistance, and toxicity. There were also the unknown long-term health effects of ART on their children (Cohan, 2003; Lyerly & Anderson, 2001).

In 1996, in developed countries, HAART, a combination drug therapy, became available to people with HIV/AIDS. This major treatment advance decreased mortality, marking a turning point in the epidemic (Hogg et al., 1997). HAART therapy offered the potential for women with HIV to live longer with chronic illness, and to continue their reproductive lives, but similar to ART, there continued to be long-term health concerns.

The idea that HIV was being seen as a chronic illness began to appear in the literature labeling people with HIV, in this case gay men, as "newly-diagnosed" compared to those with HIV as "long-standing" (Pakenham, Dadds, & Terry, 1996). Later articles on chronic illness included examples of people living with HIV, as well as other chronic conditions (Telford, Kralik, & Koch, 2006).

The research on adapting to impairment of chronic illness (Charmaz, 1995) may be useful for long-term survivors who progress from HIV to AIDS with symptoms of physical disabilities. Stages of accommodating to bodily losses and limits in relationship to self may prove helpful. Research on chronic illness challenged the concepts of "acceptance" and "denial" as stages of chronic illness as potentially detrimental to people's "re-shaping of self-identity that is fundamental when making a transition to living well with chronic illness" (Telford et al., 2006, p. 457). It is suggested that the terms of "acceptance" and "denial" are based on medical models that are not adequate for living with chronic illness in everyday experiences (Leonard & Ellen, 2008; Telford et al., 2006).

The question of people with HIV/AIDS transitioning from dying with HIV to living with it as a chronic illness has been disputed, suggesting that many people living with HIV/AIDS do not view it as chronic illness because of the uncertainty about how long the treatment will remain effective (Hoy-Ellis & Fredriksen-Goldsen, 2007).

Paterson (2001), in a metasynthesis of 292 qualitative research studies, presented a "Shifting Perspectives" model of chronic illness, challenging the linear trajectory of living with chronic illness as stages. Chronic illness is rather a managing of presentation of self where there is a dynamic shifting between wellness and illness in the foreground. Living with paradox complicates the shifting. "The major paradox of living in the wellness in the foreground perspective of chronic illness is that, although the sickness is distant, the management of the disease must be foremost; that is, the illness requires attention in order not to have to pay attention to it" (Paterson, 2001, p. 24). An example for people with HIV would be paying attention everyday to the routine of taking pills and maintaining a healthy and regular eating schedule for the physical management of HIV, while not having to pay attention to HIV daily.

People with chronic illness manage shifts of how they present themselves, depending upon their social environment and social worlds, for example, family, employment, neighborhood, and medical and social services establishments, to name a few. Leonard and Ellen (2008, p. 46) reported that "stories shift over time and across context," based on follow-up interviews with young women of color who were HIV positive and living in poverty. However, it is not clear how duration of chronic illness changes people with HIV (Pakenham et al., 1996; Paterson, 2001).

People on HAART treatment have a fragile hope for the future because of the doubts about the long-term and individual efficacy of the treatment (Vetter & Donnelly, 2006). Along with these medical uncertainties, people with HIV have questions about what it means to live physically with HIV/AIDS long term (Brashers et al., 1999). They live with shifting interpersonal relations, physical and emotional setbacks and adjustments, and fluctuations in quality of life.

Information about women's issues and concerns of living long term with HIV/AIDS can reveal what kinds of cultural notions, and medical and social interventions support or undermine women's reproductive, mothering, and living with HIV/AIDS. The discovery of the nature of women living with HIV/AIDS, particularly over time and in different social contexts, is essential to improving women's health.

METHODS

Design and Theoretical Influences

The perspectives of grounded theory (Glaser, 1978; Glaser & Strauss, 1967; Strauss, 1987; Strauss & Corbin, 1998) and feminist theory (Collins, 2000; Olesen, 2003; Smith, 1987) guided the data collection and analysis and demanded the avoidance of preconceived categories. The purpose of grounded theory is to explain variations in human activity. In grounded theory, instead of establishing a thesis to be tested in the field, "the researcher begins with an area of study and allows the theory to emerge from the data" (Strauss & Corbin, 1998, p. 12). The analyst is constantly comparing analytic products with new data to develop theoretical depictions of the forces affecting human choices and actions. Grounded theorists generally adopt the social constructionist's viewpoint of "defining the situation" as real as if it were real (Thomas & Thomas, 1970[1928]) and the social construction of reality as subjective processes (Berger & Luckmann, 1967). The symbolic interactionist's perspective on social processes includes interpreting the micro-level analysis of interaction (Mead, 1962[1934]) simultaneously with the macro-level analysis of social contexts (Strauss, 1959).

As feminists, we emulated Smith by listening to "women's experience from the woman's standpoint and explor[ing] how it is shaped in the extended relations of larger social and political relations" (1987, p. 10). Women's constructed knowledge of their life experiences was regarded as unique, in agreement with Olesen (2003). Participants were respected as central to and experts about their own stories (Collins, 2000).

Recruitment and Sampling

The sample was taken from two groups of women living with HIV ($n = 60$), one in Oakland, California ($n = 30$) and one in Rochester, New York ($n = 30$). Both groups participated in the initial study (1995–2001). The inclusion criteria are women with HIV who are living and are well enough to participate in a face-to-face interview.

Of the original 60 women, 52 women are living. Two and one-half years into this 4-year federally funded study, the author has completed 25 interviews with women from Oakland ($n = 10$) and Rochester ($n = 15$). With the continued assistance of recruiters and the recruiting protocol, it is anticipated that between 35 and 40 interviews will be completed by the end of the project.

The contact and recruiting protocol was designed on a person-by-person basis using the determinant of what is best for the potential participant. The initial contact was made by the original recruiter, provider or friend who had an established, satisfactory, trusting relationship with the potential participant. There were 33 recruiters assisting in 2 cities from a variety of medical clinics, social services agencies, and hospitals settings.

To assure integrity and success in the recruiting process, multiple training sessions were conducted with recruiters. Recruiters were paid $20 for each training session and $20 for each successful participant recruited, scheduled and interviewed. Recruiters informed participants that the purpose of the study was to investigate their experiences of reproduction, mothering, and living with HIV.

Data Collection

At the beginning of the face-to-face interview, the written informed consent was read by the potential participant who was informed anew of the purpose of the study and that they would be asked questions about their background and beliefs, and their personal and medical history. The informed consent was also available in participants' native language and the original translator was used during the interviews with two Spanish-speaking participants. Any questions were discussed and answered prior to women agreeing to participate and signing the consent form.

A $50,00 honorarium was offered in cash for participants' expertise and participation in the study and bus tokens or taxi fare in cash for transportation. Interviews were conducted in a private room of participants' choice in their residence, at their place of employment or at community facilities for medical or social services familiar to them. The data were collected between June 2005 and April 2007 with each woman interviewed in one session, except for one woman where a two-session format was used to accommodate her physical comfort. Interviews ranged from 90 minutes to 120 minutes.

This project was designed as a 10-year follow up to the original interviews. The mean time between the initial interview and the follow up was 8.2 years with a range of 5–11 years. The lower range represents participants who had sporadic use of health care, were homeless, or were not expected to live, according to recruiters. Another method of measuring long-term survivors living with HIV was considered. The mean time between participants' first HIV positive test and the follow-up interview was 14.4 years with a minimum of 8 and a maximum of 25 years.

The interviews were audio-recorded, transcribed, and analyzed using grounded theory qualitative methods (Charmaz, 2006; Glaser & Strauss, 1967; Strauss & Corbin, 1998). Qualitative research is most suitable for process-based studies and allows for participants' self-reflection concerning their actions and motives (Beardsell & Coyle, 1996; Sobo, 1995).

An interviewer-administered structured questionnaire, pre-tested with four women, was conducted at the end of the interview. A medical advisor and statistical consultant were used in the development of the questionnaire. Structured data were double-coded and double entered into Statistical Package for the Social Sciences (SPSS).

The Institutional Review Board of California State University, East Bay approved the study protocol.

It is generally accepted that behavioral research on individuals with HIV/ AIDS is beset with self-selection bias because it is limited to those who know their serostatus and are willing to talk to researchers (Siegel & Gorey, 1997). This sample is further limited since it does not represent women living with HIV from rural areas or women outside health care and social service systems. It is a close examination and conceptualization of HIV-infected women living with HIV/AIDS for over 10 years from their perspective.

Interview and Analysis Processes

Topic areas were initially developed. The usual interview started with, "Looking back over the last 10 years, can you tell me what stands out for you?" The importance of the issues of living with HIV, reproduction and mothering for each woman was part of her life story. For example, participants' concerns about communicating and being in relationship with their adult sons who they had not seen for years would prompt questions such as, "What are your concerns (plans, dreams, hopes, fears) about your relationship with your son?" Data analysis was collaborative with constant comparative and systematic processes that began with the first interview and continued throughout data collection. This process included regular meetings with grounded theory consultants at both sample sites and with research associates for shared data coding, memo writing, diagramming and theory building. Emerging themes and concepts from early interviews were then explored in more depth in ensuing interviews, but did not preclude the discovery of previously unknown themes. At varying stages of analysis, participant verification was conducted with participants (Bloor, 1997). Underlying the interview process is the means of discovery. "One must find out what the subjects themselves believe they are doing in their own terms rather than impose a preconceived or outsider's scheme of what they are doing" (Lofland, 1971, p. 4).

Participants' Characteristics

The sample ($n = 25$) was predominantly women of color (20/25), primarily African American ($n = 10$) or African ($n = 2$) with a mean age of 42 years and a range of 26–53. Slightly more than half (14/25) had an annual household income of less than \$15,000; five participants reported income of \$15,000–\$35,000, and the remaining five participants' income was \$45,000–\$99,999. Half of the participants (13/25) had subsidized housing. Thus, slightly more than half of these women were living below the poverty threshold, which is currently determined as \$23,400 for a family of five in the United States (Federal Register, 2006).

Over one third of the participants were employed (9/25) with the others not employed currently (13/25) or never employed (3/25). Almost half (11/25) had attended school since the last interview and had attained a degree (5) or certificate (4).

The majority (19/25) reported their current status as HIV positive asymptomatic (13) and symptomatic (6) and five women reported AIDS. Thus half of the women living with HIV were currently without symptoms.

Two-thirds (17/25) of the participants reported having "had a problem with addiction to drugs or alcohol." Of these 17 recovering from addiction, 5 participants (5/17) reported current drug or alcohol addiction problems.

RESULTS

"I'm Still Here"

The phrase, "I'm still here" was regularly heard in response to the questions, "What has been the biggest surprise for you over the last 10 years since I interviewed you?" Or "Looking back over the last 10 years, can you tell me what stands out for you?" A typical response was, "I'm still here." Oh, my god. I didn't think I would make it this far. I was seriously like, "Wow!" The key concept of "I'm still here" underpins what the participants talked about. The idea of still being alive and living an unexpected life permeates participants' perspectives. "I'm still here" becomes the condition for participants making sense of their life. One participant said

> Not knowing or even thinking that I would've survived –You know, that just kinda blows my mind, because, I coulda been any of women that I've seen gone.

Participants' sense of being survivors influenced their choices of mothering, taking HIV medications, disclosing their HIV status, maintaining recovery, and employment. Being long-term survivors was unexpected since participants 10 years ago spoke about their HIV as a "death sentence" (Barnes, Alforque, & Carter, 2000).

Viable but Unexpected Life

The women in this study are living what can be conceptualized as a *viable but unexpected life*. Viable has several meanings. Three themes will be used in presenting this analysis.

Surviving Outside the Womb

It is fascinating to consider this definition of viable as used to describe a fetus that can survive outside the womb. It is intriguing that female long-time survivors of HIV are birthing a new life that can survive outside their former lives before they learned their diagnosis, lives that may have involved substance use, prostitution, homelessness, domestic violence, or other social issues. It suggests a new life, and the ability of participants to survive on their own, living independently, despite the burdened journey.

> The most joyful thing, oh (sigh) is that I lasted this long. Yeah. That I lasted this long. "Cause any time, I coulda just gave up and just – let go and went back to that ol' life. And say, "Forget it, 'cause it's gon' happen anyway." You know. So, I think the most joyous thing to me is that I'm still hangin'. I'm still hangin'. and I'm gonna be hangin' tomorrow and the day after. (laughing).

Normalcy

Making a viable life suggests normalcy, fitting in, and life as part of a recognized group of individuals, such as the mother of a child, a volunteer in a social service agency to help others, a paid worker at a well-thought-of organization such as a school or a medical office, and a person with a place to live that she can call her own. Participants were keeping appointments, going back to work, attending school and college, seeking employment and eating regularly, which is often a prerequisite for maintaining the HIV medication protocol. Participants were developing a life style of managing the side effects of medication, maintaining sobriety, feeding their kids, going to events for their kids, and going to work. An example of developing normalcy is how one participant re-defined what she used to think was fun when she was an injecting drug user and what she now defines as going to the park, movies, or camping with her kids.

> This is what fun is all about. I'm thinkin' sittin' in some empty, abandoned house, you know, waitin' on somebody to bring me somethin' – it was fun? No. This here is fun. Me an' my kids, we go campin', the movies, all that was great, you know? An' continue to be great, hopefully.

Participants spoke of the tensions between the joys and challenges of the unexpected life, giving particular emphasis to issues pertaining to mothering. Mothering was described as life sustaining with consequences as depicted by this respondent.

> I don't like the challenges that go along with it [mothering], but I'm very proud of being a mom. I'm glad I had my kids, now. 'Cause if I didn't have my kids and I hadda deal with this illness, I would not be here. I would not. My kids – they give me a reason for being. I coulda gave up when I first got very ill, but, I always wanted to see my babies grow up. I always wanted to see how they were gonna be when they grow up, so I fought more. And then I fought more, and I continue on fighting, and, to this day, I'm still fighting, you know.

The joys and challenges of mothering included experiences of attempting to gain contact with children that participants had given up for adoption, making up for lost time with kids, having to put children in foster care through mothers relapsing from drug recovery or a son's destructive behavior and self-mutilation. Here is an example of a mother's experience of the tensions between the challenges and joys.

> This is another one [child] who, uh, got taken [adopted] because of my drug addiction, in 1988. So next month he'll be 18, and I just feel that's been hard for me because, that's my kid – that's how I feel. And at that time, you know it wasn't the right time. But that's something I still deal with, because I feel a lot of guilt, behind that (voice breaking, crying) and I want to see him really bad (crying).

She was hopeful that she would reconnect with him. She had initiated procedures with a social worker that could assist her son in the event that he might attempt to find her, his birth mother.

Typically, participants who were in recovery and who had missed mothering their young children due to substance abuse, spoke of the challenges of raising their children who were living with them. Mothering was avoiding patterns of parenting that they disliked about their own childhood experiences. Mothering was encouraging, advising, watching, and monitoring and playing with their children, and letting their children know they love them.

(tears, crying) My mother never show any love. I'm forty-eight years old and I think I've heard my mother say "I love you" once to me. I think that's the reason why I feel wrapped up in my kids, 'cause I want them to know that I love them!

Life Worth Doing

Another dimension of living as a long-time survivor was in making the unexpected life count, to make it worth doing, possibly leaving a legacy. For some, this "worth doing" was making up for the guilt of lost mothering time with their children.

"I think I'm a good mother (pause of several seconds, tears, crying) but I think what it means is I try too hard to please, to make up for what I did." It can also be helping others, particularly other HIV positive women, by being a peer mentor, advocate, educator, or counselor. Often through this outreach work, long-time survivors earned social status, and an identity different from what they had before being diagnosed. This identity could perhaps afford them income, education, commendation, recognition among their peers and their community of friends, their children's friends, and, if they had disclosed publicly, to their community and larger family of origin. One participant said

I like helping other woman, because I know how it is to break from one habit to another habit, it is not easy just to cross that line, to know that you can be somebody – you are somebody, you have some qualities no matter, where've you been.

Tensions of Living a Viable but Unexpected Life

Tensions abound among categories that dimensionalize the concept of living a viable but unexpected life with HIV as a chronic illness. The tensions of living with dying; of looking healthy and being scared of being hospitalized; of experiencing a downward spiral that initiates fear of dying with each new or reoccurring symptom; of between being in drug recovery and relapsing. Other conditions that participants shared were issues of disclosure to children, potential intimate partners, and co-workers that influenced maintaining relationships and avoiding isolation.

DISCUSSION/CONCLUSIONS

An unexpected life with HIV challenges participants as long-term survivors to live with a chronic illness, developing a viable life that is different from their pre-diagnosed life. It involves a life of defining normalcy in everyday experiences and building a legacy of an unexpected life worth living. The results demonstrate how the participants living long term with HIV changed them, building on Pakenham et al. (1996), and Paterson (2001). Participants made changes from their former lives; for example, from dependency on substance use to returning to college or employment or seeking employment. Participants were living with hope for a future sustained by their everyday experiences of mothering or, in some cases, grand-mothering and living for their children and grandchildren. This hope was more fragile for some, particularly those women seeking to find and reconnect with children they had given up for adoption.

Chronic illness for study participants was not talked about in terms of "denial" or "acceptance" or even endurance but was more the notion of regaining a life that they had presumed would be short-lived. Participants were living with uncertainties and tensions, as mentioned above. Some of these uncertainties were centered on HIV, such as the possibility of downward spiraling that initiates fear of dying. Other tensions were focused on drug recovery, and finding employment and economic security.

The results support the notion of managing presentation of self as a dynamic shifting between wellness and illness in the foreground and living with paradoxes that complicate the shifting (Paterson, 2001). However, there was less evidence of the participants' process of adapting to stages of disabilities as suggested by Charmaz (1995). Larger longitudinal and follow-up studies of women living more than an average of 14 years from a variety of geographical locations may prove informative.

Future research could attempt to investigate what Charmaz (2002) refers to as the silences in the stories of research participants who live with chronic illness. What are the elements of women's long-term living with HIV that they are not talking about or that they have not yet found the words or means of expressing? For example, one study participant kept "silent" about her daughter's suicide. Prior to the interview with this participant, the recruiter had alerted the author of the daughter's suicide. In the interview that took place in her home, the participant spoke of her children in detail, including sharing photographs of them, but not her deceased daughter. The point is well taken that "The voice of suffering and the void of silence alert us to the perils of imposing narratives on often fragmented, elusive stories participants struggle to tell" (Charmaz, 2002, p. 323).

At this phase in the analysis, there are many other ideas under exploration. For example, participants' spiritual beliefs were more prominent in the original study with ideas of God as comforter, protector, and ultimate authority in reproductive decisions. Was the initial study more representative of crises times? Are participants' current lives less crises laden? How much credit is given to medical advances and treatment and how much to God's will? How are these reconciled? How is that expressed in daily life? What continues to influence participants keeping their HIV status a secret or revealing it? What effect does keeping secrets have on participants?

Participants' issues and concerns of living with HIV/AIDS identify what kinds of cultural notions, and medical and social interventions support or undermine women's mothering and long-term living with HIV/AIDS. The results offer knowledge pertaining to HIV positive women's quality of life. This study informs and can enhance current medical and social services for women in recovery and enhance women's abilities to manage uncertainties and fears. Counseling techniques for women with HIV could be further developed for assistance with women's education and gaining employment and housing for a more stable economic future. The findings have policy implications for implementing innovative programs on mothering skills, assistance in re-uniting families, and community-based medical and social services to promote optimal support and services for HIV positive women and their children.

ACKNOWLEDGMENTS

This research was funded by the National Institutes of General Medical Sciences grant GM 48135. The content is solely the responsibility of the author and does not necessarily represent the official views of the National Institute of General Medical Sciences or the National Institutes of Health. An earlier draft was present at the American Sociological Association Annual Meeting, New York, August 12, 2007.

The author wishes to thank the women who shared their experiences and their reflections; also the consultants Sheigla Murphy, Maggie Kearney, Susan Taylor-Brown, Monica Bill Barnes, and Craig Sellers for their contributions to data analysis and valuable feedback; and Audrey Alforque Thomas for statistical analysis and literature review, and Parul Baxi for research support.

REFERENCES

Barnes, D. B., Alforque, A., & Carter, K. (2000). Like I just got a death sentence: Conditions affecting women's reactions to being told their HIV antibody test results and the impact on access to care. *Research in the Sociology of Health Care, 18,* 3–33.

Barnes, D. B., & Murphy, S. (2009). Reproductive decisions for women with HIV: Motherhood's role in envisioning a future. *Qualitative Health Research* (accepted for publication).

Beardsell, S., & Coyle, A. (1996). A review of research on the nature and quality of HIV testing services: A proposal for process-based studies. *Social Science and Medicine, 42*(5), 733–743.

Berger, P. L., & Luckmann, T. (1967). *The social construction of reality: A treatise in the sociology of knowledge.* Garden City, NY: Doubleday.

Bloor, M. (1997). Techniques of validation in qualitative research: A critical commentary. In: G. Miller & R. Dingwall (Eds), *Context and methods in qualitative research* (pp. 37–50). London: Sage.

Brashers, D. E., Neidig, J. L., Cardillo, L. W., Dobbs, L. K., Russell, J. A., & Haas, S. M. (1999). "In an important way, I did die": Uncertainty and revival in persons living with HIV or AIDS. *AIDS Care, 11*, 201–219.

Centers for Disease Control and Prevention. (1985). Recommendations for assisting in the prevention of perinatal transmission of human T-lymphotropic virus type III/ lymphadenopathy-associated virus and acquired immunodeficiency syndrome. *Morbidity and Mortality Weekly Report, 41*, 1–23.

Centers for Disease Control and Prevention. (1993). 1993 revised classification system for HIV infection and expanded surveillance case definition of AIDS among adolescents and adults. *Morbidity and Mortality Weekly Report, 34*, 721–732.

Charmaz, K. (1995). The body, identity, and self: Adapting to impairment. *Sociological Quarterly, 36*(4), 657–680.

Charmaz, K. (2002). Stories and silences: Disclosures and self in chronic illness. *Qualitative Inquiry, 8*(3), 302–328.

Charmaz, K. (2006). *Constructing grounded theory: A practical guide through qualitative analysis.* London: Sage.

Cohan, D. (2003). Perinatal HIV: Special considerations. *International AIDS Society, 11*(6), 200–213.

Collins, P. H. (1994). Shifting the center: Race, class, and feminist theorizing about motherhood. In: M. B. Zinn & B. T. Dill (Eds), *Women of color in US society.* Philadelphia: Temple University Press.

Collins, P. H. (2000). *Black feminist thought: Knowledge, consciousness, and the politics of empowerment* (2nd ed.). New York: Routledge.

Connor, E. M., Sperling, R. S., Gelber, R., Kiselev, P., Scott, G., O'Sullivan, M. J., VanDyke, R., Bey, M., Shearer, W., Jacobson, R. L., Jimenez, E., O'Neill, E., Bazin, B., Delfraissy, J. F., Culnane, M., Coombs, R., Elkins, M., Moye, J., Stratton, P., & Balseley, J. (1994). Reduction of maternal infant transmission of human immunodeficiency virus type 1 with zidovudine treatment. *New England Journal of Medicine, 331*(18), 1173–1180.

Federal Register. (2006, January 24). *Federal Register, 71*(15), 3848–3849.

Fleming, P. L., Lindegren, M. L., Byers, R., Hammett, T., Harris, N., Schulte, J., & Janssen, R. (2002). Estimated number of perinatal HIV infections, U.S., 2000, July. Poster session [TuPeC4773] presented at XIV Annual International AIDS Conference, Barcelona, Spain.

Glaser, B. G. (1978). *Theoretical sensitivity: Advances in the methodology of grounded theory.* Mill Valley, CA: The Sociology Press.

Glaser, B. G., & Strauss, A. L. (1967). *The discovery of grounded theory: Strategies for qualitative research.* New York: Aldine De Gruyter.

Hogg, R. S., O'Shaughnessy, M. V., Gatric, N., Yip, B., Craib, K., Schecter, M. T., & Montaner, J. S. (1997). Decline in deaths from AIDS due to new antiretrovirals. *Lancet*, *349*, 1294.

Hoy-Ellis, C. P., & Fredriksen-Goldsen, K. I. (2007). Is AIDS chronic or terminal? The perceptions of persons living with AIDS and their informal support partners. *AIDS Care*, *19*, 835–843.

Leonard, L., & Ellen, J. M. (2008). "The story of my life": AIDS and "Autobiographical Occasions". *Qualitative Sociology*, *31*, 37–56.

Levine, C., & Dubler, N. N. (1990). HIV and childbearing: Uncertain risks and bitter realities: The reproductive choices of HIV-infected women. *The Milbank Quarterly*, *68*(3), 321–351.

Lofland, J. (1971). *Analyzing social settings*. Belmont, CA: Wadsworth.

Lyerly, A. D., & Anderson, J. (2001). Human immunodeficiency virus and assisted reproduction: Reconsidering evidence, reframing ethics. *Fertility and Sterility*, *75*(5), 843–858.

Mead, G. H. (1962). *Mind, self, and society* ((Original work published 1934)). Chicago: The University of Chicago Press.

Olesen, V. (2003). Feminisms and qualitative research at and into the millennium. In: N. K. Denzin & Y. S. Lincoln (Eds), *The landscape of qualitative research: Theories and issues* (pp. 332–397). Thousand Oaks, CA: Sage.

Pakenham, K. I., Dadds, M. R., & Terry, D. J. (1996). Adaptive demands along the HIV disease continuum. *Social Science and Medicine*, *42*(2), 245–256.

Paterson, B. L. (2001). The shifting perspectives model of chronic illness. *Journal of Nursing Scholarship*, *33*(1), 21–26.

Personal conversation. (2008). HIV activist (name withheld) who marched with ACT-UP in San Francisco in 1990, February 28.

Siegel, K., & Gorey, E. (1997). HIV-infected women: Barriers to AZT use. *Social Science and Medicine*, *45*(1), 15–22.

Smith, D. E. (1987). *The everyday world as problematic: A feminist sociology*. Boston: Northwestern University Press.

Sobo, E. J. (1995). HIV testing and wishful thinking. In: E. J. Sobo (Ed.), *Choosing unsafe sex: AIDS-risk denial among disadvantaged women* (pp. 140–156). Philadelphia: University of Pennsylvania Press.

Sterling, T. R., Lyles, C. M., Vlahov, D., Astemborski, J., Margolick, J. B., & Quinn, T. C. (1999). Sex differences in longitudinal human immunodeficiency virus type-1 RNA levels among seroconverters. *Journal of Infectious Diseases*, *180*, 666–672.

Strauss, A. (1959). *Mirrors and masks: The search for identity*. Glencoe, IL: Free Press.

Strauss, A. L. (1987). *Qualitative analysis for social scientists*. New York: Cambridge University Press.

Strauss, A. L., & Corbin, J. (1998). *Basics of qualitative research: Techniques and procedures for developing grounded theory* (2nd ed.). Thousand Oaks, CA: Sage.

Telford, K., Kralik, D., & Koch, T. (2006). Acceptance and denial: Implications for people adapting to chronic illness: Literature review, August. *Journal of Advanced Nursing*, *55*(4), 457–464.

Thomas, W. L., & Thomas, D. S. (1970). Situations defined as real are real in their consequences. In: G. P. Stone & H. A. Farberman (Eds), *Social psychology through symbolic interaction* (pp. 154–155). Waltham, MA: Ginn-Blasdell (original work published 1928).

Vetter, C. J., & Donnelly, J. P. (2006). Living long-term with HIV/AIDS: Exploring impact in psychosocial and vocational domains. *Work*, *27*, 277–286.

SECTION 4:
MENTAL HEALTH

PHYSICIANS AS ADVOCATES FOR THEIR PATIENTS: DEPRESSION TREATMENT IN PRIMARY CARE

Ashley A. Dunham, Teresa L. Scheid and William P. Brandon

ABSTRACT

This chapter explores how primary care physicians deliver mental health treatment for Medicaid patients in one county in the United States, and how treatment may have changed after HMO enrollment with a mental health carve-out. We utilize Lipsky's theory of street-level bureaucracy to better understand how primary care physicians treat Medicaid patients for depression and what types of insurance arrangements support or inhibit that treatment. Exploratory interviews with 20 physicians revealed that the patient's status as a non-voluntary client, service system barriers and physicians' commitment to treatment caused them to bear primary responsibility for the majority of depression care. Physicians were willing to act as advocates for their clients and viewed such advocacy as ethical given the lack of mental health parity. In general, primary care physicians were not familiar with new policies dictating mental health carve-outs for Medicaid patients, nor were they concerned with how mental health care was reimbursed for their patients. However, they were willing to provide mental health care even if they were not reimbursed. Physicians rely upon

Care for Major Health Problems and Population Health Concerns:
Impacts on Patients, Providers and Policy
Research in the Sociology of Health Care, Volume 26, 141–165
Copyright © 2008 by Emerald Group Publishing Limited
All rights of reproduction in any form reserved
ISSN: 0275-4959/doi:10.1016/S0275-4959(08)26007-2

medication management to treat depression, and reimbursement plays a role in the amount of time spent with patients and in the coding used for the visit. Lipsky's (1980) theory of street-level bureaucracy provides a useful framework for understanding how physicians will act as advocates for their clients in the face of structural as well as resource constraints on health care.

INTRODUCTION

Despite the fact that mental health care registered the greatest increase (153%) in the general medical care service sector in the United States from the early 1990s to 2003 (Wang et al., 2006), there has been relatively little research on exactly how primary care physicians practicing in the United States respond to the mental health needs of their clients. In general, primary care physicians believe they are able to respond more appropriately to the mental health needs of their patients in integrated settings involving other mental health care providers (Gallo et al., 2004; Lin et al., 1997). However, the perceived availability of mental health resources, the stigma associated with mental illness, gender, ethnicity, and co-existing medical conditions of their patients and illness severity also affect the willingness and ability of primary care physicians to treat mental illness (Borowsky et al., 2000; Croghan, Schoenbaum, Sherbourne, & Koegel, 2006). Recent qualitative studies regarding primary care treatment of depression have focused on patient responses rather than physician responses (Okello & Neema, 2007; Switzer, Wittink, Karsch, & Barg, 2006). This chapter uses information from exploratory interviews with primary care physicians in one county in the Southeastern United States to examine what kind of mental health treatment they provide and what types of insurance support or inhibit that treatment. The study site had undergone a recent change to a mandatory mental health carve-out for Medicaid[1] enrollees that eliminated primary care reimbursement for mental health treatment. Consequently, this data also allows us to examine how reimbursement mechanisms affect primary care physician treatment of mental health as well as how physicians respond to the mental health needs of Medicaid patients.

Health care carve-outs are best understood as a form of health insurance that excludes certain services such as mental health from prepaid health plan arrangements. Its rationale is that carve-outs will reduce the moral hazard of specific services by having specialists manage those benefits

(Frank, Huskamp, McGuire, & Newhouse, 1996, p. 227). The services provided under a carve-out are managed separately and have distinct budgets, provider networks, and incentive arrangements (Frank, McGuire, & Newhouse, 1995). Mental health carve-outs affect the behavior of health care providers by changing financial incentives and creating forces that are intended to modify treatment based on payment (Kassirer, 1995). Although some research assumes the physician to be a wealth maximizer (Inkelas, 2001), other studies also support information dissemination and physician knowledge as stronger determinants of clinical practice patterns than reimbursement arrangements (Sturm & Wells, 1998). Hoff and McCaffrey (1996) found that doctors felt new payment schemes interfered with the relationship they had with patients.

The manner in which physician behavior and patient relationships will be affected by financial incentives will depend on the specific carve-out arrangement. When mental health care is carved out and reimbursed on a fee-for-service basis and primary care is reimbursed on a fee-for-service basis, both the primary care providers and mental health care providers have the incentive to increase business volume as long as the marginal cost of care is less than the marginal revenue received from providing that care. Therefore, the primary care provider is likely to refer patients to mental health if they are perceived to be time-consuming or problem cases (Goldberg, 1999) which might prevent the physician from maximizing his/her income. This model supports some best practice guidelines for primary care physicians to treat less severe mental illness in their practices, particularly when less time-consuming efforts are acceptable, such as the use of psychotropic drugs to manage depression (Elkin et al., 1989; Kupfer et al., 1992; Pincus et al., 1998).

Conversely, when mental health care is carved out and primary care is capitated (as was the case in our study site) primary care providers have a clear incentive to identify and move mental health care out of their practices and into the mental health sector, because mental health care is not included in their capitated rate. Although this shifting of patients from primary care to mental health may result in more efficient and effective mental health treatment for some patients (Katon et al., 1995), this arrangement does not serve to support the primary care treatment of less severe depression, which can be effective when implemented properly (Wells et al., 2000; Wells et al., 2004).

This chapter is based on an exploratory study which sought to understand primary care treatment of depression, how primary care physicians viewed mental health carve-outs, and whether such carve-outs had any effect on how they dealt with the mental health needs of their Medicaid clients. We found Lipsky's (1980) theory of street-level bureaucracy was useful in explaining physician behavior; we therefore begin with an overview of this perspective. We then move to a consideration of the findings, and a more thorough discussion of the ways in which we found physicians acted as advocates in order to meet the mental health needs of their patients.

PHYSICIANS AS STREET-LEVEL BUREAUCRATS

Most theory relevant to public policy has described physician behavior either through an economic explanation of responses to reimbursement and the labor-leisure tradeoff (Pauly, 1981; Reinhardt, 1999) or sociological theory exploring professional dominance (Freidson, 1970; Haug, 1988; Navarro, 1988; Wolinsky, 1988). Traditional economic theory assumes that physicians will manage their time so as to maximize their own utility (including wealth and other factors that contribute to a person's happiness). Even with the constraints imposed by a variety of factors (market for services, government, time available, relationship with patients, etc.) this theory assumes that physicians will typically behave so as to maximize the overall net income they can receive from medical practice (Zweifel & Breyer, 1997). However, tests of this model at the empirical level remain limited, and other economic models that include additional factors provide better explanations of physician behavior (Reinhardt, 1999).

Sociological studies of professional dominance (Hafferty & McKinlay, 1993) have focused on how new forms of bureaucratic control over medical practice (i.e., managed care) have affected the professional status of physicians. Recent research on the changing status of medical professionals lends support to Freidson's (1984) argument that the professions continue to exercise control of their work (Griffiths & Hughes, 1999; Hafferty & McKinlay, 1993; Weiss & Fitzpatrick, 1997). For example, Griffiths and Hughes (1999) found a negotiated division of labor between managers and physicians in the British National Health Service (NHS), and that decisions about clinical care still relied upon medical expertise. Weiss and Fitzpatrick (1997) found that while physicians (GPs) were in fact conforming to principles of cost containment, clinical autonomy was preserved.

Understanding physician response to the mental health needs of their clients must also be placed within the context of the asymmetrical nature of the doctor–patient relationship (Clark & Mishler, 1991; Maeside, 1991; Maynard, 1991; Waitzken, 1989). Differentials in power are due to more fundamental of imbalance in medical knowledge (Silverman, 1987). Physicians not only have the professional authority to diagnosis illness and to prescribe treatment (Maynard, 1991); they also control the process by which patients receive information (Clark & Mishler, 1991). Medical language and the "voice of medicine" can overlook and/or downplay patients' concerns, or the "voice of the lifeworld" (Katz, 1984; Mishler, 1984). With increased external control over medicine (i.e., mechanisms to manage care), physicians have even less time to attend to patient's mental health needs.[2]

Even though physicians are considered public servants, little theoretical research actually links physician behavior to this role (Checkland, 2004; McDonald, 2002). One approach that fills this void is that of "street-level bureaucracy" (Lipsky, 1980). Lipsky defines street-level bureaucrats as "public service workers who interact directly with citizens in the course of their jobs, and who have substantial discretion in the execution of their work" (Lipsky, 1980, p. 3). Typical street-level bureaucrats are public school teachers, police officers, and social workers. However, in the context of delivering care to patients enrolled in public health programs such as Medicaid, primary care physicians can also be considered street-level bureaucrats. Using the concept of street-level bureaucracy expands the theory-base for explaining how physicians actually behave in their day-to-day interactions with patients, particularly in relation to their framing and response to the mental health problems of their patients.

The theory of street-level bureaucracy (Lipsky, 1980, p. 82) predicts that front-line public servants develop "routines and simplifications" to help deal with the pressures associated with demand that outstrips supply. Primary care physicians face internal pressures when they work under the constraints of managed care; patient satisfaction is affected by the length of time spent with physicians (Gross, Zyzanski, Borawski, Cebul, & Stange, 1998), physicians perceive that managed care organizations dictate limits on office visits (Mechanic, McAlpine, & Rosenthal, 2001), and physicians feel a "hassle and burden" of providing care under managed arrangements along with a feeling of disconnect from the processes of policy implementation (Chaudry, Brandon, Thompson, Clayton, & Schoeps, 2003, p. 37). As a result, physicians develop "routines" to deal with the demand for quality regardless of the supply of time. These "routines and simplifications" of "street-level" bureaucrats then become the unwritten policies actually carried out by their organizations.

Street-level bureaucrats are asked to be more than gatekeepers and rationers of public service. They are also expected to be advocates, that is, to use their knowledge, skill, and position to secure for clients the best treatment within the constraints of the bureaucracy. This is particularly true for physicians, who even as early as medical school take the Hippocratic Oath to offer the best care possible to their patients. Most enter the field hoping to help others, but quickly learn that many of their actions are ineffective. This ineffectiveness is exacerbated by the responsibility to deliver services efficiently and limit expenditures, an example being when a primary care physician wishes to treat mental health but does not receive any reimbursement for this service. Given resource constraints (a capitated arrangement) and a mental health carve-out, physicians may not be able to deliver what they consider "best practice." Lipsky (1980) suggests that professionalism may be a possible solution to service dilemmas faced by street-level bureaucrats performing advocacy roles. Physicians, by virtue of their professional status, are less accountable to organizational constraints. Physicians have been able to preserve their clinical autonomy as decisions about clinical care are primarily based upon medical expertise (Griffiths & Hughes, 1999; Weiss & Fitzpatrick, 1997).

Associated with the advocacy role of physicians is the Medicaid patient's non-voluntary status. Clients are considered non-voluntary when they have relatively no choice about where they obtain necessary health services. Medicaid patients are viewed as non-voluntary because their inability to afford health insurance elsewhere leaves them with relatively few choices among the limited number of physicians who accept Medicaid. This status creates a relationship between the patient and physician where the physician has nothing to lose by not satisfying their patients. Instead, physicians will try to manage a large volume of patients and their complaints, but will not change policy in response to client dissatisfaction (Lipsky, 1980). Sociological research on doctor–patient interactions has also found that physicians do not address the deeper roots of client's health care problems; "social change is not a therapeutic option" (Waitzken, 1989, p. 227). Instead physicians help clients to adjust and attempt to manage clients' complaints so as to not appear difficult or unresponsive to their needs.

In addition to this problematic interaction, the patient is also acting with limited information and typically lacks the knowledge necessary to complain about inadequate treatment (Mishler, 1984). Under a carve-out where the primary care physician is not reimbursed for mental health care, this relationship offers a choice: should physicians interpret the policy in their own best interest by maximizing income and not treating mental health problems? Or should they act on the patient's behalf by disregarding state-level policy and effectively treating mental health care problems in the primary care office? Lipsky (1980) predicts that physicians would attempt to treat the patient effectively by acting as their advocate. However, with their "corporate" responsibilities (the carve-out precluding mental health in the physicians' capitated income) and the Medicaid patient's non-voluntary status, physicians would do their best to manage a large number of clients, and either provide quick and costless treatment (write a quick prescription),[3] or refer them to public mental health services that are supposedly available through the carve-out.

Although Lipsky (1980) often refers to physicians in his text, very little research has used his theory to interpret physician behavior. McDonald (2002) used the theory of "street-level bureaucracy" to explain the behavior of physicians when new policies were implemented in Britain's NHS. In the 1990s, the NHS assessed new technologies being implemented in Primary Care Groups against the criterion of clinical cost-effectiveness, specifically to assist in the allocation of scarce health care resources. McDonald (2002) studied the process of service planning related to coronary heart disease and found that the decision-making process for how to best treat coronary heart disease was markedly at odds with the rational health economic approach. Instead of focusing on agency objectives and technical solutions to allocate resources, the physicians used their own discretion and attempted to satisfy a large number of patients using an expeditious workload philosophy. Because approximately 90% of episodes of care in the NHS begin and end in primary care, the opportunities for top-down control are limited, leaving physicians with considerable discretion as to how they perform. The physicians examined in her study did not follow agency objectives, instead reacting to perceived problems and treating each patient according to his/ her particular needs. Her findings suggest that general practitioners will continue to exercise individual discretion rather than respond to central guidance. McDonald's conclusion is not only consistent with theories of professional dominance, but it also supports Lipsky's (1980) conception of the street-level bureaucrat as the policy maker rather than the policy implementer.

Checkland (2004) also used the ideas of Lipsky to analyze practice-level responses to the implementation of National Service Frameworks (NSFs) in Britain's NHS, which specified detailed models of service provision that health care providers were expected to follow. Checkland (2004) examined the general practitioners' implementation of NSFs in relation to the successful execution of purely clinical practice guidelines established by medical societies (in particular, the British Hypertension Society). Checkland (2004) discovered that even when primary care practices had a positive track record of implementing clinical practice guidelines, the NSFs had very little practical impact. Because the NSFs were perceived as too complicated, the physicians (acting as street-level bureaucrats) did not view them as aiding in the processing of clients. Many of the physicians explained that they only adopted those guidelines that would "make the job easier," not those such as NSFs which involved more than one actor and contributed to an already excessive workload. The evidence from Checkland's (2004) study indicates that the NSFs were only being implemented to a limited extent, and that real policy was being "enacted" on the ground by general practitioners who ignored official priorities. This finding lends support to Lipsky's (1980) idea that the behavior of street-level bureaucrats becomes the "de facto" policy of organizations.

RESEARCH OBJECTIVES

Our chapter focuses on the important question of how primary care physicians respond to the mental health needs of their Medicaid clients, particularly when mental health reimbursement mechanisms are changed, and therefore addresses the context within which policy changes are worked through and enacted. More specifically, we examine whether physicians do in fact act as advocates for their clients regardless of reimbursement, and how physicians acting as street-level bureaucrats have shaped the various ways in which Medicaid clients receive mental health care.

This exploratory research was guided by four central questions. First, how do primary care physicians interpret (i.e., understand) state policy relevant to the financial reimbursement of mental health for their Medicaid clients? Second, to what degree do primary care physicians serve as advocates for their clients by treating mental health problems? Third, what barriers exist to the provision of mental health care? Fourth, how does the patient's status as a non-voluntary client affect the physician's treatment of mental health problems?

METHODS

Study Site

An urban county in the Southeastern United States was selected for qualitative research to gain a deeper understanding of how primary care physicians treat Medicaid patients for depression, what kind of treatment they provide, and what types of insurance arrangements support or inhibit that treatment. This county provided an excellent research setting because of the implementation of mandatory Medicaid enrollment in risk-bearing HMOs (health maintenance organizations) in 1996.[4]

This Medicaid managed care project, which carved out mental health and prescription drugs from capitated arrangements with primary care gatekeepers, offered an opportunity to explore physician interpretation of a specific state policy and its effect on primary care treatment of mental health problems. We focused on depression because of its high prevalence, particularly in the primary care setting (Kessler et al., 1994) and the economic burden of the illness, estimated at 83.1 billion in 2000 (Greenberg et al., 2003).

Sample

A list of 300 physicians was compiled from the state Medical Society and the state Medical Board, and a letter was sent soliciting their participation in a survey examining the treatment of depression in primary care. The letter included an endorsement from the local Medical Society. A total of 20 physicians (9 women and 11 men) responded to the letter and all were interviewed by the senior author in the summer and fall of 2005. Appendix contains the questions used in the semi-structured interview (Morse & Field, 1995). Prior to the interviews drafts of interview questions were reviewed for content validity by two primary care physicians who were in practice in the study county, and their suggested revisions were incorporated. All participants gave informed consent before answering any questions and the project was approved by the University IRB. Interviews lasted from 20 minutes to 1 hour and physicians were encouraged to express other thoughts and feelings not specifically asked in the interview questions.

The average age of physicians interviewed was 43 years old. Two African-American physicians participated in the interviews and 18 were Caucasian. There was an average of 8.25 physicians in their practice: two practiced internal medicine; three, pediatrics; and the remainder, family medicine. An average of 25% of their patient population was on Medicaid, and a little over half ($n = 12$) were practicing in the county during mandatory Medicaid HMO enrollment.

Data Analysis

The interviews were recorded and transcribed by the first author, and reviewed by the second author. The data was analyzed by N5 (Richards, 2000), a program that allows coding and comparison of interview text files. Eleven different themes that emerged during the analysis of the data:

1. Causes of depression
2. Effects of reimbursement arrangements
3. Reasons primary care physicians treat depression
4. Patient acceptance of counseling referrals for depression
5. Alternative coding for depression visits to ensure reimbursement
6. How training affects depression treatment
7. Communication with mental health providers
8. Mental health services available to Medicaid patients
9. Specific comments on mental health carve-outs
10. Financial incentives
11. Barriers to "best practice."

Reports were created from these categories, and interview information was analyzed and organized into the four dimensions stated in the Objectives. Two of the authors and a third party with qualitative interviewing expertise analyzed the node information. After an initial 85% agreement between the first two authors and third party, additional discussions yielded 100% agreement on the analysis.

RESULTS

Primary Care Physician's Interpretation of State Policy and Medicaid Reimbursement for Mental Health

In general, the primary care physicians who were interviewed expressed a lack of knowledge regarding mental health reimbursement arrangements for their patients. This lack of knowledge was consistent among the majority of those interviewed; most were unwilling to use their time to examine how their patient's insurance reimbursed mental health. The physicians repeatedly used the terminology "it would all balance out in the long run," meaning reimbursement from all their patients would provide enough to satisfy their needs to maximize wealth, even if they did not receive payment for some of their services because of inadequate or nonexistent health insurance. This feeling was particularly true for those physicians in salaried arrangements.

> I'm not paid solely on claims. As long as my paycheck is pretty good at the end of the year, I'm not looking at the day to day billing. Somebody else might be a lot more focused on how much they were billing. I just treat patients as efficiently as possible, and hope we all turn out all right in the long run. I'm sure I treat a lot that we never see payment for.

However, similar sentiments were expressed by those who were not salaried, embodied by the following statement.

> I never had a financial bent. If there were a few who didn't pay, I didn't worry much about it. The insurance didn't dictate how I treated patients. I found out that if I tried to let the insurance decide how I treated, I spent more resources doing that than taking care of the patients. If you try to beat the insurance companies, you end up losing in the long run.

All the physicians expressed a willingness to take care of a patient's mental health even if they were not reimbursed for that service. Many said that ignoring a patient's mental health problems would cost them more in unnecessary office visits, because the patient would return repeatedly with somatic complaints until the mental health issues were addressed. After being asked if their behavior changed in response to the Medicaid mental health carve-out, one physician said

> I continued to treat mental health, even when the mental health was not included in the capitated rate. Even if you didn't [treat mental health], they [the patient] would still call you because they couldn't get mental health. They would end up coming back with somatic complaints, so it wasn't worth trying to refer them out for mental health conditions that I could treat in the office.

This quote makes specific references to mandatory Medicaid HMO enrollment with capitated arrangements and the mental health carve-out: the policy change of interest. Primary care physicians were paid a monthly capitated rate per Medicaid patient during mandatory HMO enrollment rather than traditional fee-for-service reimbursement. These capitated rates paid for all primary care delivery *except* for mental health and prescription drugs.

Twelve out of the 20 physicians interviewed were practicing primary care in the study county during mandatory Medicaid HMO enrollment. There were mixed recollections of how the carve-out affected their willingness and ability to treat mental health, with some physicians remembering their behavior changing in response to the carve-out and others not recalling any change in the way they treated their Medicaid patients for mental health.

One physician who continued to treat mental health said, "I still treated my patients, because I knew they didn't have a good place to go and they didn't want to go outside of my office for mental health." In addition to providing an example of physician response during a mental health carve-out, this statement represents two significant barriers to Medicaid patients with mental health problems: the physician perception of an overall lack of high quality mental health services available to Medicaid patients and the patient's unwillingness to seek treatment for mental health outside of the primary care office. As well as the primary care physician's belief that they are responsible for both the patient's mental and physical health, these two barriers may partially explain why primary care physicians continued to treat mental health in their office while their monthly capitated reimbursement did not include mental health.

However, there were physicians who expressed a change in their behavior with the implementation of the carve-out.

> I would say that I didn't spend any time on that issue [depression], and tried to refer out the majority of my patients. That's why I try to divorce myself from a patient, of what type of insurance they have because it would really drive you crazy.

Although some physicians recollected a response to the carve-out, others did not. Based on the qualitative recollections, definitive conclusions regarding how physicians respond to a change in policy cannot be drawn. Many physicians appeared unaware of the change in policy, and even those who were aware did not necessarily change their behavior. The physicians explained their lack of change with several factors, including a perceived lack of mental health resources in the area, the stigma associated with mental illness, and the physician's confidence in their ability to treat depression. These overall issues with mental health treatment were also reflected in other physician responses to mental health insurance arrangements, such as the deliberate miscoding of mental health visits to guarantee reimbursement. This topic is covered in the next section, along with Lipsky's idea of the street-level bureaucrat as advocate.

The Beliefs and Willingness of Primary Care Physicians to Serve as Advocates for Their Patients by Treating Mental Health

Any action by a primary care physician to recognize mental health problems and either treat, or refer a client to mental health care, involves some advocacy on behalf of their clients. As mentioned in the previous section, most physicians believed they were capable of treating most cases of depression. The physicians were very specific as to which mental health conditions they felt comfortable treating, and which were beyond their scope of practice. Across the board, primary care physicians felt comfortable treating depression among all populations, with the exception of one pediatrician who was concerned with the liability associated with prescribing certain antidepressant medications to children.

Similarly, the majority of physicians interviewed expressed the inability to separate the mind from the body, as this quote illustrates.

> I would love for everyone to be able to see that I cannot separate the mind from the body, and if I don't treat them for depression, they are going to be coming into my office with all these other things. It's much more rewarding to get to the heart of the matter and treat depression … It would be nice to be able to code for exactly what is wrong, not what I know they'll pay for.

All the physicians expressed the necessity in treating mental health in the primary care office, because the patient was unwilling to seek mental health services from a different provider, or the services available to them were difficult to obtain and their insurance was often inadequate.

Lipsky (1980) argues that street-level bureaucrats put the clients' needs first through their advocacy position, evidenced by the primary care physician's need to treat depression. But many times their advocacy position conflicts with other corporate responsibilities, such as the need to efficiently process clients. This efficiency would not include providing treatment for services that provide no financial remuneration to the physicians or their employer. These interview findings suggest that physicians continued to serve as advocates and treated their patients for depression, but in a way that continued to be efficient for them and their employer. Efficient depression treatment in the primary care office typically involves only pharmacologic management, due to a lack of office visit time and a lack of residency training for psychotherapy (Frank, Huskamp, & Pincus, 2003). By only treating patients with antidepressants primary care physician were able to satisfy both their advocacy needs and corporate responsibilities, even if this may have meant less than ideal care for their patients.

When asked if they treated current patients for mental health regardless of available reimbursement, primary care physicians whose patients had private insurance stated that they provided depression treatment and creatively coded the visit in order to receive reimbursement, thereby satisfying their need to serve as the patient's advocate but still serve their own financial interests. Twelve out of the 20 physicians specifically stated that coding for physical complaints rather than mental complaints was an ethical response to the lack of parity in mental health coverage. One physician stated

> Some patients, in order for their mental health visit to get paid, require that I not bill them for mental health problems. To bypass this, I find something else wrong, for example low back pain, and bill them for this although I am treating the emotional complaint instead. Most insurers have specific mental health benefits, but they're easy to get around because you can just code for the symptom, not the diagnosis.

Physicians repeatedly expressed the willingness and necessity of treating both mental and physical health, particularly with the Medicaid patients. Most of the primary care physicians believed that the mental health resources available to their Medicaid patients were so flawed that the only choice they had with less severe mental illness was to treat in their office. The sentiment surrounding Medicaid mental health services is embodied in the following quote.

> There aren't that many [providers] who take Medicaid. They have to go to the mental health center. They [mental health] are apparently overwhelmed and busy. People [patients] complain all the time. We don't get notes back from the mental health providers. By and large you don't know what is going on. They won't necessarily see the same provider. It's like a black box.

Because of the non-voluntary status of the patient and their lack of available resources, the physicians are left with primary responsibility for mental health issues such as depression that they believe can be effectively treated in the primary care office. However, with large caseloads often seen in primary care offices, time with patients is limited. This limitation, as well as other financial and policy-related barriers, affects the type of care these physicians provide. In order to provide what they learned was adequate depression care without spending unavailable amounts of time, pharmacologic care with little or no counseling was the most common treatment cited. Depending on reimbursement mechanisms, physicians may have responded with longer and more frequent visits. However, their care typically consisted of medication management, which is often considered inadequate for effective depression treatment (Wells et al., 2004). In addition to treatment limitations caused by inadequate time during the patient visit and a lack of residency training in psychotherapy, other barriers prevented optimal treatment. These barriers are discussed in the next section.

Barriers That Prevent the Primary Care Physicians from Providing High Quality Depression Care

The primary care physicians interviewed for this study discussed several financial and policy barriers that prevented them from providing the highest quality depression care for their Medicaid patients. Limited time during an office visit was of major concern for those primary care physicians expressing an inability to adequately treat depression in their office.

> I only have 15 minutes, and I am treating them for so many other things. Talking to them about weight loss, diabetes, and then I have to squeeze in a depression screening.

The majority of those physicians interviewed recommended a three-pronged approach to depression treatment: lifestyle changes such as exercise and weight loss, referral to outside psychotherapy and antidepressant medications. This approach is evidenced in the following quote from a family physician.

> I like to treat it with three different arms. I think medications can help people. Studies show that medications can be extremely effective in treating depression. Physical activity can be helpful, and talking with a counselor. I like my patients to do all three. It increases their odds of successful treatment. If they have bad insurance or Medicaid, I try to play the counselor role, but I am not as effective.

Patient resistance to treatment, particularly delivered outside of the primary care office, was also a concern. According to the physicians interviewed, only about 10% of patients who were referred to an outside source for depression treatment actually followed through with the referral. The combination of physician reluctance to refer and patient failure to visit mental health providers when referred left the primary care physician treating the majority of their patients for depression. The physicians also felt unable to control or lessen the chronic stressors that were often a part of depression, such as financial and social problems. These stressors were often cited during the interviews as a major cause of depression among the Medicaid population. For example:

> What I notice more are just the lingering effects of chronic social problems. It just beats people down over time. Chronic stress, mostly financial. That circumstance is only exacerbated by biochemistry malfunction and heredity. These [external] stressors cannot be changed, so pharmacologic treatment is the only option.

With these inescapable problems, even if the physician was able to provide counseling to the patient, total relief from stressors that worsen the depression would not be attainable. However, there were also physicians who believed that body biochemistry was the main cause of depression. This genetic predisposition, coupled with external factors, caused depression to surface in most individuals.

> The main cause that I see is true endogenous depression. There are just chemicals in the brain and people who benefit from us altering that. Also you have the prolonged stress. So you have the external situations coupled with long-standing serotonin depletion.

There was a general consensus of a lack of available psychiatric resources, particularly for the Medicaid population. The physicians interviewed articulated their concern regarding insufficient resources for Medicaid patients.

> I can get angry with a patient who doesn't go see their cardiologist, because I know a cardiologist is available to them and will get a note back to me in a timely fashion. With mental health, it's not the same. Those providers just aren't available. The only people that I really insist follow through with the referral are those who are beyond my scope, and may require more than one medication or are suicidal.

Most in the group interviewed were aware of the lack of psychotherapy, and would often play the "counseling role" if necessary. However, limited office visits and lack of training creates less than ideal situations. This quote from a physician sums up the general sentiment regarding mental health.

> There [are] so many problems it's hard to know where to start. It would be helpful if insurance companies would be a lot more willing to provide reimbursement [to primary care physicians] for more common mental health problems. It would be helpful if patients had easier access to therapists without a higher copay. I don't know what therapists are good. It's hard to come up with a good name for someone to see, especially if they are on Medicaid.

With a lack of mental health resources, limited time for office visits and patient resistance to referrals, primary care physicians stated that they were often the sole providers of depression care. Because of a lack of training, they were left treating less severe depression in their office with antidepressants and little or no counseling. This care may have been seen as inadequate for many patients, but allowed the physicians to meet their responsibility as the patient's advocate as well as their "corporate responsibilities" of efficient care delivery. The primary care physicians may have believed this behavior fulfilled their role as an advocate, but it left the patient with less than adequate care for depression (Wells et al., 2004). Lipsky's theory of street-level bureaucracy explains that physicians rationalize this less than adequate care because of the Medicaid patient's status as a non-voluntary client.

The Medicaid Patient's Status as a Non-Voluntary Client and its Effect on Primary Care Depression Treatment

Lipsky defines the non-voluntary clients as those who are "force[ed] to seek assistance through public agencies or not seek assistance at all" (Lipsky, 1980, p. 54). Medicaid clients are viewed as non-voluntary because they have no means other than the State for securing health insurance. As a result, their choice of providers is limited, particularly for mental health. Lipsky asserts that the providers who serve these clients have nothing to lose in failing to satisfy them. For that reason, clients often receive less than adequate services because of their lack of control over who is delivering the services to them and the quality of those services. Lipsky also suggests that the providers have nothing to lose by not satisfying their clients because there is a relatively inexhaustible supply of Medicaid patients. This supply would permit constant replacement of those Medicaid patients who were unhappy with their depression treatment with those who were relatively happy with the limited services they could receive from primary care physicians.

Even with primary care physicians having nothing to lose by failing to satisfy their patients covered by Medicaid, the majority of primary care physicians expressed concern about delivering sub-standard depression care. This concern represents an overall primary care physician consensus in being responsible for the large majority of a patient's health care, including mental health issues (deGruy, 1996). However, there was a clear understanding among the physicians that Medicaid patients had very little to no choice regarding mental health services. This circumstance created a predicament for primary care physicians. How could they continue to be advocates for their patients by referring them to what they perceived to be an inadequate mental health facility? A solution for most was to provide limited treatment in their office. A pediatrician surveyed declared

> We are in the front lines. It's like ADD [attention deficit disorder]. If we sent everyone out [for depression treatment] to a specialist it would take them too long to get them through the system. In a perfect world we would have quick and immediate mental health services available, but that's just not how it works.

Of those physicians surveyed, the majority of them believed that primary care treatment of depression can be effective, and some believed they were just as effective as mental health professionals.

> If they are functional, not psychotic or suicidal, then they're [Medicaid patients] probably going to do as well with me as they would with any psychologist or psychiatrist

> I could get them in to see. God help you if you're suicidal because you're going to have to wait two weeks [to see a psychiatrist]. I have always treated them in my office because the system is so bad.

So the physicians were able to satisfy their predicament by treating the majority of depression in their office, knowing that the non-voluntary status of the patients limited both the resources available to them and the influence that the patients may have on treatment. With non-voluntary status, patients are willing to accept less than satisfactory care because of their inability to seek care elsewhere. If the primary care physicians had believed their Medicaid patients had a choice of providers and a realistic chance of receiving alternative care if they were dissatisfied with the public mental health system, their reactions might be different. They might feel more comfortable referring out mental health treatment because services would be available. The physicians might also have reacted differently with a different population such as the privately insured, who were more important to retain and had a voluntary relationship with the physician.

In summary, the physicians repeatedly expressed concern about the lack of services available to the Medicaid patients. This concern regarding lack of services was compounded by the non-voluntary nature of Medicaid patients, allowing less than adequate care to take place due to the consequences of limited number and range of services available. One physician said

> The predominant people [patients] I have are Medicaid and the predominant provider is the behavioral health center [public facility]. The main complaint is that they can't get an appointment. So de facto we end up managing them.

However, most physicians believed that pharmacologic care was effective enough to satisfy their patient advocacy role; it was the default service provided to those Medicaid patients who had inadequate alternatives. One physician stated

> You try your best to get them to go to counseling, and they just won't go or they can't get into mental health [the public facility for Medicaid patients]. You try to explain to them that doing counseling and medication is best, but they still need to be treated. You can't withhold the medication just because they can't go to counseling. Usually the medication is your best bet to get [the depression] under control.

DISCUSSION

We first summarize our major findings. In general, primary care physicians were not familiar with new policies dictating mental health carve-outs for

Medicaid patients, nor were they concerned with how mental health care was reimbursed for their patients. However, they were willing to provide mental health care even if they were not reimbursed, and were comfortable prescribing anti-depressants for depression. If necessary, physicians were willing to code diagnoses in a manner that would generate reimbursement; 60% of those interviewed were willing to code for somatic complaints rather than mental illness if that would allow treatment to be reimbursed. Physicians were willing to act as advocates for their clients and viewed such advocacy as ethical given the lack of mental health parity.

The physicians we interviewed were also concerned with the lack of mental health services and resources for their clients, and were also constrained in their ability to provide mental health care by limited office time and lack of training in psychotherapy. They provided what care they could by prescribing anti-depressants. Because Medicaid patients are non-voluntary clients (i.e., they have no other means for obtaining care and limited choice of providers), physicians were able to rationalize their behavior in offering these patients what physicians believed to be less than optimal care. Lipsky's (1980) theory of street-level bureaucracy provides a unique framework for understanding how physicians will act as advocates for their clients in the face of structural as well as resource constraints on health care.

While the findings are important, data limitations should be noted. The data were collected from a small number of primary care physicians in one area of the United States. In addition, self-selection bias was introduced when the only physicians interviewed were those who responded to the request for participation, most likely representing those physicians more interested in mental health issues than their colleagues who did not volunteer to take part. Interviewing the physicians rather than observing actual behavior also introduces interview bias; more unobtrusive data gathering techniques in their work settings may have given a more realistic picture of their response to the mental health needs of their clients. Furthermore, we have little insight into how physicians came to recognize and therefore treat mental health problems, although the interviews do demonstrate that physicians are concerned with the mental health needs of their clients and believe that most cases of depression can be treated in primary care settings with anti-depressants. Physicians also expressed support for psychotherapy, and were frustrated by resource constraints which limited their ability to serve as counselors, or to refer their patients out for counseling. Physicians also were aware that chronic stressors were a major source of depression for their Medicaid patients. Finally, the time that lapsed between the implementation of new Medicaid policy and the physician interviews may limit the physician's ability to accurately recall their response to new policy.

Further research should examine a larger, systematic sample of physicians operating under diverse financial reimbursement structures in order to determine under what financial conditions are physicians willing to advocate for their clients. Lipsky (1980, p. 56) draws on Freidson (1970) to suggest that "doctors in private practice can also neglect patients if there is a restricted supply of professionals, but they become much more soliticitous when patients have medical alternatives upon which to draw." Will physicians play an advocacy role for voluntary clients who have some choice of providers? Under what conditions do they play an advocacy role for non-voluntary clients? Does the advocacy role for non-voluntary clients extend to other types of illness or behavioral problems (e.g., substance abuse)? To what degree do shortages of providers affect physician relations with patients? These are just a few of the questions that need to be addressed.

Our research also provides a new perspective of physician behavior. Viewing primary care physicians as street-level bureaucrats allows us to speculate how changes in policy may affect care-giving practices. In a system that strictly follows corporate policy (in this case, Medicaid policy), the mental health carve-out with a capitated primary care arrangement would encourage the use of specialty mental health services to treat all mental health care, even for those who could be treated by a primary care physician. However, the primary care physicians interviewed for this study did provide office-based treatment for depression. The official carve-out policy may have encouraged referral for all mental health care, but the de facto policy was different. While reimbursement is an important factor in determining behavior (Feldman, Ong, Lee, & Perez-Stable, 2006), physicians serving as street-level bureaucrats will only enact policy that allows them to serve their role as both as an advocate and a bureaucrat with corporate responsibilities. This unofficial policy is adjusted in an attempt to meet the needs of a patient population with inadequate resources, where the demand for services for Medicaid patients exceeds the supply of physicians willing to provide those services. In summary, using new theory to interpret physician behavior provides a unique contribution to an already existing body of literature that aims to predict how primary care physicians respond to their patients' mental health needs.

NOTES

1. Medicaid is a joint federal/state program that provides health care benefits to groups of low-income people, some who may have no medical insurance or inadequate medical insurance.

2. We agree with Mishler (1984, p. 11) and a large body of sociological theory that illnesses are constructed, and it is likely that mental health problems will not be addressed unless the patient takes a fairly pro-active role in calling attention to these problems.

3. This behavior was documented in a study by Weilburg, O'Leary, Meigs, Hennen, and Stafford (2003)where primary care physicians were prescribing antidepressants in ways that were unlikely to be effective across a broad spectrum of patients.

4. The authors acknowledge that there is a significant time gap between the implementation of a mental health carve-out and when this research was conducted. This research was part of a larger project examining all facets of primary care, and we acknowledge the limitations created by the physician's ability to accurately recall the effects of a policy change on their behavior.

ACKNOWLEDGMENTS

We would like to thank the primary care physicians who participated in this study, and the Metrolina Medical Foundation for supporting this research.

REFERENCES

Borowsky, S. J., Rubenstein, L., Meredith, L., Camp, P., Jackson-Triche, M., & Wells, K. B. (2000). Who is at risk of nondetection of mental health problems in primary care? *Journal of General Internal Medicine, 15*(6), 381–388.

Chaudry, R. V., Brandon, W. P., Thompson, C. R., Clayton, R. S., & Schoeps, N. B. (2003). Caring for patients under Medicaid mandatory managed care: Perspectives of primary care physicians. *Qualitative Health Research, 13*(1), 37–56.

Checkland, K. (2004). National service frameworks and UK general practitioners: Street-level bureaucrats at work? *Sociology of Health and Illness, 26*(7), 951–975.

Clark, J. A., & Mishler, E. G. (1991). Attending to patients' stories: Reframing the clinical task. *Sociology of Health and Illness, 14*, 344–372.

Croghan, T. W., Schoenbaum, M., Sherbourne, C. D., & Koegel, P. (2006). A framework to improve the quality of treatment for depression in primary care. *Psychiatric Services, 57*(5), 623–630.

deGruy, F. (1996). Mental health care in the primary care setting. In: M. S. Donaldson, K. D. Yordy, K. N. Lohr & N. A. Vanselow (Eds), *Primary care: America's health in a new era*. Washington, DC: National Academy Press.

Elkin, I., Shea, M. T., Watkins, J. T., Imber, S. D., Sotsky, S. M., Collins, J. F., Glass, D. R., Pilkonis, P. A., Leber, W. R., Docherty, J. P., et al. (1989). National institute of mental health treatment of depression collaborative research program: General effectiveness of treatments. *Archives of General Psychiatry, 46*(11), 971–982.

Feldman, M., Ong, M. K., Lee, D. L., & Perez-Stable, E. J. (2006). Realigning economic incentives for depression care at UCSF. *Administration and Policy in Mental Health and Mental Health Services Research, 33*(1), 34–38.

Frank, R. G., Huskamp, H. A., McGuire, T. G., & Newhouse, J. P. (1996). Some economics of mental health "carve-outs". *Archives of General Psychiatry, 53*, 933–937.

Frank, R. G., Huskamp, H. A., & Pincus, H. A. (2003). Aligning incentives in the treatment of depression in primary care with evidence-based practice. *Psychiatric Services, 54*(5), 682–687.

Frank, R. G., McGuire, T. G., & Newhouse, J. P. (1995). Risk contracts in managed mental health care. *Health Affairs, 14*(3), 50–64.

Freidson, E. (1970). *Profession of medicine: A study of the sociology of applied knowledge.* New York: Harper & Row.

Freidson, E. (1984). The changing nature of professional control. *Annual Review of Sociology, 19*, 1–20.

Gallo, J. J., Zubritsky, C., Maxwell, J., Nazar, M., Bogner, H. R., Quijano, L., Syropoulos, H. J., Cheal, K. L., Chen, H., Sanchez, H., Dodson, J., & Levkoff, S. E. (2004). Primary care physicians evaluate integrated and referral models of behavioral health care for older adults: Results from a multi-site effectiveness model (PRISM-E). *Annals of Family Medicine, 2*(4), 305–309.

Goldberg, R. J. (1999). Financial incentives influencing the integration of mental health care and primary care. *Psychiatric Services, 50*(8), 1071–1075.

Greenberg, P. E., Kessler, R. C., Birnbaum, H. G., Leong, S. A., Lowe, S. W., Berglund, P. A., & Corey-Lisle, P. K. (2003). The economic burden of depression in the United States: How did it change between 1990 and 2000?. *Journal of Clinical Psychiatry, 64*, 1465–1475.

Griffiths, L., & Hughes, D. (1999). Talking contracts and taking care: Managers and professionals in the British national health service internal market. *Social Science and Medicine, 44*, 1–13.

Gross, D., Zyzanski, S., Borawski, E., Cebul, R., & Stange, K. (1998). Patient satisfaction with time spent with their physician. *Journal of Family Practice, 47*, 133–137.

Hafferty, F. W., & McKinlay, J. B. (Eds). (1993). *The changing medical profession: An international perspective.* Oxford University Press: New York.

Haug, M. R. (1988). A re-examination of the hypothesis of physician deprofessionalization. *Milbank Quarterly, 66*(2), 48–56.

Hoff, T., & McCaffrey, D. P. (1996). Adapting, resisting, and negotiating: How physicians cope with organizational and economic change. *Work and Occupations, 23*, 165–189.

Inkelas, M. (2001). Incentives in a specialty carve-out. *RAND Graduate School*, Santa Monica, University of California, Los Angeles.

Kassirer, J. P. (1995). Managed care and the morality of the marketplace. *New England Journal of Medicine, 333*, 50–52.

Katon, W., Von Korff, M., Lin, E., Walker, E., Simon, G. E., Bush, T., Robinson, P., & Russo, J. (1995). Collaborative management to achieve treatment guidelines. Impact on depression in primary care. *Journal of the American Medical Association, 273*(13), 1026–1031.

Katz, J. (1984). *The silent world of doctor and patient.* New York: The Free Press.

Kessler, R. C., McGonagle, K. A., Zhao, S., Nelson, C. B., Hughes, M., Eshleman, S., Wittchen, H. U., & Kendler, K. S. (1994). Lifetime and 12 month prevalence of DSM-III-R psychiatric disorders in the United States. Results from the national comorbidity survey. *Archives of General Psychiatry, 51*(1), 8–19.

Kupfer, D. J., Frank, E., Perel, J. M., Cornes, C., Mallinger, A. G., Thase, M. E., McEachran, A. B., & Grochocinski, V. J. (1992). Five-year outcome for maintenance therapies in recurrent depression. *Archives of General Psychiatry, 55*(7), 645–651.

Lin, E. H., Katon, W., Simon, G. E., Von Korff, M., Bush, T., Rutter, C. M., Saunders, K. W., & Walker, A. (1997). Achieving guidelines for the treatment of depression in primary care: Is physician education enough? *Medical Care, 35*(8), 831–842.

Lipsky, M. (1980). *Street-level bureaucracy: Dilemmas of the individual in public services.* New York: Russell Sage Foundation.

Maeside, P. (1991). Possibly abusive, often benign, and always necessary: On power and domination in medical practice. *Sociology of Health and Illness, 13,* 545–561.

Maynard, D. (1991). Interaction and asymmetry in clinical discourse. *American Journal of Sociology, 97*(2), 448–495.

McDonald, R. (2002). Street-level bureaucrats? Heart disease, health economics and policy in a primary care group. *Health and Social Care in the Community, 10*(3), 129–135.

Mechanic, D., McAlpine, D. D., & Rosenthal, M. (2001). Are patient's office visits with physicians getting shorter? *New England Journal of Medicine, 344*(3), 198–204.

Mishler, E. G. (1984). *The discourse of medicine: Dialectics of medical interviews.* Norwood, NJ: Ablex Publishing Corporation.

Morse, J. M., & Field, P. A. (1995). *Qualitative research methods for health professionals* (2nd ed.). Thousand Oaks: Sage Publications, Inc.

Navarro, V. (1988). Professional dominance of proletarianization? *Milbank Quarterly, 66*(2), 57–75.

Okello, E. S., & Neema, S. (2007). Explanatory models and help-seeking behavior: Pathways to psychiatric care among patients admitted for depression in Mulago Hospital, Kampala, Uganda. *Qualitative Health Research, 17*(1), 14–25.

Pauly, M. V. (1981). *Doctors and their workshops: Economic models of physician behavior.* Chicago: University of Chicago Press.

Pincus, H. A., Tanielian, T., Marcus, S. C., Olfson, M., Zarin, D. A., Thompson, J., & Zito, J. M. (1998). Prescribing trends in psychotropic medications: Primary care psychiatry, and other medical specialties. *Journal of the American Medical Association, 279*(7), 526–531.

Reinhardt, U. (1999). The economist's model of physician behavior. *Journal of the American Medical Association, 281*(5), 432–437.

Richards, L. (2000). *Using N5 in qualitative research.* Australia: QSR International Pty Ltd.

Silverman, D. (1987). *Communication and medical practice: Social relations in the clinic.* London: Sage Publications.

Sturm, R., & Wells, K. B. (1998). Physician knowledge, financial incentives and treatment decisions for depression. *The Journal of Mental Health Policy and Economics, 1,* 89–100.

Switzer, J. F., Wittink, M. N., Karsch, B. B., & Barg, F. K. (2006). Pull yourself up by your bootstraps: A response to depression in older adults. *Qualitative Health Research, 16*(9), 1207–1216.

Waitzken, H. (1989). A critical theory of medical discourse: Ideology, social control, and the processing of social context in medical encounters. *Journal of Health and Social Behavior, 30*, 220–239.

Wang, P. S., Demler, O., Olfson, M., Pincus, H. A., Wells, K. B., & Kessler, R. C. (2006). Changing profiles of service sectors used for mental health care in the United States. *American Journal of Psychiatry, 163*(7), 1187–1198.

Weilburg, J. B., O'Leary, K. M., Meigs, J. B., Hennen, J., & Stafford, R. S. (2003). Evaluation of the adequacy of outpatient antidepressant treatment. *Psychiatric Services, 54*(9), 1233–1239.

Weiss, M., & Fitzpatrick, R. (1997). Challenges to medicine: The case of prescribing. *Sociology of Health and Illness, 19*, 297–327.

Wells, K. B., Sherbourne, C., Schoenbaum, M., Duan, N., Meredith, L., Unutzer, J., Miranda, J., Carney, M. F., & Rubenstein, L. V. (2000). Impact of disseminating quality improvement programs for depression in managed primary care. *Journal of the American Medical Association, 283*(2), 212–220.

Wells, K. B., Sherbourne, C., Schoenbaum, M., Ettner, S., Duan, N., Miranda, J., Unutzer, J., & Rubenstein, L. (2004). Five-year impact of quality improvement for depression: Results of a group-level randomized controlled trial. *Archives of General Psychiatry, 61*(4), 378–386.

Wolinsky, F. D. (1988). The professional dominance perspective, revisited. *Milbank Quarterly, 66*(2), 33–47.

Zweifel, P., & Breyer, F. (1997). *Health economics* (2nd ed.). New York: Oxford University Press.

APPENDIX. INTERVIEW QUESTIONS

Demographics and Practice Information

1. Race?
2. Gender?
3. Age?
4. Specialty area?
5. How many physicians are in your practice?
6. How many years have you been practicing medicine?
7. What percent of your patient population is covered by Medicaid?
8. What percent of your patient population is uninsured?

Questions Related to Depression

9. What is the approximate prevalence of depression among your patient population?
10. Are there any particular populations where you see more depression?
11. What do you feel is the main cause of depression?

12. What are some of the challenges you see in effectively diagnosing depression?
13. Usually, what are the next steps you take after a diagnosis?
14. Does the patient's insurance (or lack of) have an effect on how you treat their depression? If so, how?
15. Does your practice follow strict guidelines related to the treatment of depression?
16. Do you often make referrals for depression treatment, or do you treat the patients in your office?
17. Can you think of any other policy related issues that affect your ability to effectively treat depression?
18. Have you ever heard of "mental health carve-outs?"
19. Were you practicing in Mecklenburg County when the Medicaid program instituted mandatory managed care enrollment (between 1996 and 1997)?
20. If so, did you realize that the HMO was not including mental health treatment in the capitated rates that physicians received?
21. How do these mental health carve-outs affect your ability to treat depression in your office?
22. What are some of the patient-related issues that affect depression treatment?
23. Related to depression, can you think of anything else that may have an effect on your treatment decisions?

Questions Related to the Nature and Scope of Primary Care

24. Why did you choose to enter a primary care field?
25. Would you say that your style of practicing medicine is more affected by your residency training, or by your current surroundings (your current practice, colleagues, etc.)?

SOCIAL SUPPORT AND THE USE OF MENTAL HEALTH SERVICES AMONG ASIAN AMERICANS: RESULTS FROM THE NATIONAL LATINO AND ASIAN AMERICAN STUDY

Ethel G. Nicdao, Seunghye Hong and
David T. Takeuchi

ABSTRACT

Objective: *Our study examines the association between social support and use of mental health services in Asian American men and women. Specifically, we report on the association between types of social support and types of health services used (general medical care and specialty mental health care).*

*   ***Method:*** *We use data from the National Latino and Asian American Study, a nationally representative survey of the US household population of Latino and Asian Americans. Our present study is based on data from the sample of Asian Americans (N = 2,095).*

Care for Major Health Problems and Population Health Concerns:
Impacts on Patients, Providers and Policy
Research in the Sociology of Health Care, Volume 26, 167–184
Copyright © 2008 by Emerald Group Publishing Limited
All rights of reproduction in any form reserved
ISSN: 0275-4959/doi:10.1016/S0275-4959(08)26008-4

Results: Overall, our findings suggest that Asian Americans use general medical care services more than specialty mental health care. Our findings also showed variations in levels of social support, and the use of health services among different Asian subgroups (Vietnamese, Filipino, Chinese, and Other Asian) and nativity status (US-born versus foreign-born Asians). Specific types of social support influenced the use of specialty mental health care services, while other types of social support inhibited use of specialist services.

Conclusion: Compared to using generalist services, Asian Americans demonstrated lower rates of using specialist services. Our results emphasize the importance of considering other social factors to explain between group differences as well as factors contributing to the underutilization of specialty mental health services by Asian Americans.

SOCIAL SUPPORT AND THE USE OF MENTAL HEALTH SERVICES AMONG ASIAN AMERICANS

Evidence exists that social support, defined as "the gratification of a person's basic social needs through social interaction with others" (Kaplan, Cassel, & Gore, 1977), serves as a protective factor for people facing various life stressors (Cobb, 1976) and can buffer individuals from stressful life events and ongoing negative life strains (Thoits, 1982, 1986). Social support has been shown to assist people in maintaining their health during difficult life situations (Turner, Pearlin, & Mullan, 1998).

Few studies explore the association between social support and mental health among ethnic minority populations. Results from a recent study on African Americans indicate that social support was associated with fewer depressive symptoms (Lincoln, Chatters, & Taylor, 2005). Another recent study on Latinos showed that social support was strongly associated with self-rated mental health (Mulvaney-Day, Alegria, & Sribney, 2007). A study on Vietnamese immigrants showed that social support from nonkin was associated with a reduction in depression scores over time (Gellis, 2003).

Using social support theory as a framework for our study, we draw from the works of social support researchers (Cobb, 1976; Thoits, 1984) to answer the question: Does level of social support influence the use of mental health services among Asian Americans? Using data from the National Latino and Asian American Study (NLAAS), we test the influence of social support on use of mental health services. We hypothesize that individuals with high levels of social support are better able to cope with major life changes and events and therefore less likely to use mental health services. Conversely, those with little or no social support may be more vulnerable to life changes and events and therefore more likely to use mental health services.

SOCIAL SUPPORT, ASIAN AMERICANS AND MENTAL HEALTH SERVICES

Social support tends to come from family, friends, and co-workers; social needs come in the form of socioemotional aid or instrumental aid. Socioemotional aid includes affection, sympathy, understanding, acceptance, and esteem. Instrumental aid includes advice, information, help with responsibilities, and financial aid (Thoits, 1982). Some research studies indicate that individuals who possess a strong social support system experience less distress and are least likely to seek help, while those with little or no social support are more vulnerable to distress experiences (Gellis, 2003; Thoits, 1995). This same line of research also suggests that individuals can be buffered from negative life events if they can retain a high level of social support (Thoits, 1982).

Studies on social support among Asian Americans are growing. Research findings suggest that the benefit of social support is seen more in terms of how individuals perceive the availability of social support rather than in utilizing social support resources. In other words, knowledge and awareness of having social support may reduce stress more than seeking actual help (Taylor et al., 2004).

Among ethnic minority groups, the use of mental health services has been well-documented (Herrick & Brown, 1998; Takeuchi & Kim, 2000). Research studies have shown that generally, ethnic minority groups access and use public mental health services to varying degrees (Barreto & Segal, 2005; Hu, Snowden, Jerrell, & Nguyen, 1991; Takeuchi & Kim, 2000). A recent study conducted by the National Center for Health Statistics provides more compelling evidence of mental health disparities among ethnic minorities. In particular, compared to US born adults, foreign-born adults benefit positively from many health measures despite limited access to health care services. For mental health indicators, US born and foreign-born adults were equally likely to experience serious psychological distress (Dey & Lucas, 2006).

A study on the use of public mental health services among ethnic populations showed Asians and Hispanics using less emergency and inpatient services but more outpatient care than Whites, while Blacks used more emergency services and less outpatient care (Hu et al., 1991). For Asian Americans, studies have found that Asians underutilize mental health services and utilize services in varying rates (Abe-Kim et al., 2007; Okazaki, 2000; Yamashiro & Matsuoka, 1997). For example, one study revealed that US-born Asian Americans used health services at a higher rate than immigrant Asians and service use patterns were linked to nativity and generation status (Abe-Kim et al., 2007). Another study compared 6-month utilization of mental health services by Asian Americans and found that the most outpatient encounters were experienced by East Asians and Filipinos. Moreover, East Asians and Filipinos spent a considerable amount of time in outpatient services, and used the most inpatient care (Barreto & Segal, 2005). Some researchers have attributed various factors to explain the underutilization of mental health services including: cultural beliefs, lack of trust in the mental health system, lack of comfort with Western methods, stigma and shame, acculturation, and family support (Herrick & Brown, 1998).

RESEARCH METHODS

Data

NLAAS is a nationally representative survey of the US household population of Latino and Asian Americans. The NLAAS study is the first national epidemiological survey of Latinos and Asian Americans which aims to assess lifetime and 12-month prevalence of mental illness and mental health service use, to estimate the relation of social position (neighborhood cohesion, social standing), environmental context (social networks and social cohesion), and psychosocial factors, and to compare prevalence with non-Latino whites and African Americans. Our present study was based on data from the sample of Asian Americans in the NLAAS project. Participants were non-institutiona-lized people of Asian ancestry who were 18 years of age or older, and resided in any of the 50 states and Washington DC. A total of 2,095 Asian American participants were recruited between May 2002 and November 2003. Written informed consent was obtained for all participants and all study procedures and protocols were approved by Institutional Review Boards at University of Washington, Cambridge Health Alliance, Harvard University, and the University of Michigan. For a detailed description of the NLAAS protocol and sampling methods, see (Heeringa et al., 2004).

Measures

Sociodemographic variables included gender, age, education, marital status, employment status, and income. *Nativity* measured whether the respondent was born in the US (US-born) or outside of the US (foreign born). The variable *Asians* included four subgroups: Vietnamese ($N = 520$), Filipino ($N = 508$), Chinese ($N = 598$), and Other Asians ($N = 467$).

Social support was measured based on questions related to social networks. We used both support and harmony to measure the larger concept of "social support." However, support and harmony are different continuous variables and were used separately in the analyses. *Family support* included three questions and was based on a scale scored from 1 (most) to 5 (least): (1) How often do you talk on the phone or get together with family or relatives who do not live with you? The five response categories range from "Most every day (1)" to "Less than once a month (5)." (2) How much can you rely on relatives who do not live with you for help if you have a serious problem? (3) How much can you open up to relatives who do not live with you if you need to talk about your worries? For the second and the third questions, four response categories range from "A lot (1)" to "Not at all (4)." *Family support* was based on a sum of scores from the three questions, so that higher scores indicate a higher degree of support than lower scores. *Friend support* was measured based on the questions: (1) How often do you talk on the phone or get together with friends? (2) How much can you rely on friends for help if you have a serious problem? (3) How much can you open up to your friends if you need to talk about your worries? The scale and response categories for *friend support* were the same as those used for family support. *Friend support* was also based on a sum of scores so that higher scores indicate a higher degree of support than lower scores. *Family harmony* asked respondents: (1) How often do your relatives or children make too many demands on you? (2) How often do your family or relatives argue with you? *Friend harmony* included the questions: (1) How often do your friends make too many demands on you? (2) How often do your friends argue with you? The two questions for family harmony and friend harmony was based on a scale scored from 1 (often) to 4 (never). *Family* and *friend harmony* was based on summed scores to indicate that higher scores meant higher degree of harmony.

K10 Psychological Distress is a scale developed for use in epidemiological surveys and measures outcomes following treatment for common mental health disorders. The scale asked the following: "During the last 30 days, about how often did you ..." (1) feel depressed? (2) feel so depressed that nothing could cheer you up? (3) feel hopeless? (4) feel restless or fidgety?

(5) feel so restless that you could not sit still? (6) feel tired out for no good reason? (7) feel that everything was an effort? (8) feel worthless? (9) feel nervous? (10) feel so nervous that nothing could calm you down.

Use of services (*generalist and specialist*) was assessed with the question "In the past 12 months, did you go to see [provider on list] for problems with your emotions, nerves, or your use of alcohol or drugs?" Three types of services were assessed for the study: (1) specialty mental health care (psychiatrist, psychologist, other mental health professional, or hotline); (2) general medical care (general practitioner, nurse, occupational therapist, other health professional, or any other medical doctor; and (3) any services (social worker, counselor, religious or spiritual adviser) and alternative services (herbalist, doctor of Oriental medicine, chiropractor, spiritualist, internet support group, or self-help group). This variable was dichotomously coded ($0 =$ none, $1 =$ at least once) [Abe-Kim et al., 2007].

Methodology

Our main analyses consisted of a series of multivariate logistic regression to examine the associations between social support (i.e., support and harmony, separately) and 12-month mental health related service use (i.e., generalist and specialist) because 12-month service uses behave like binary outcome variables. For our initial models, we used a stratified sample by including the nativity variable in our model and conducted analyses using separate models for each of the Asian subgroups. Because of our smaller sample sizes, models for each of the Asian subgroups allowed us to conduct only partial analyses, controlling for fewer variables. We then compared the results for the different Asian subgroups to assess any variations. Logistic regression analyses were conducted using the SUrvey DAta ANalysis (SUDAAN) software system to adjust for sample weights and sample design effects. We reported weighted percentages, means, and standard errors when presenting sociodemographic characteristics of the sample.

FINDINGS

Table 1 shows the sociodemographic characteristics for the sample. The majority of respondents were foreign born (77%). The mean for seeing a generalist was higher than the mean for seeing a specialist. The higher scores for family and friend support indicate that respondents had higher degrees of support than family or friend harmony.

Table 1. Sociodemographic Characteristics for Asian American Sample ($N = 2,095$).

	Unweighted N	Weighted Percentage/Mean	SE (%)
Gender			
Men	998	47.45	1.22
Women	1097	52.55	1.22
Nativity			
US-born	454	23.06	3.16
Foreign-born	1639	76.94	3.16
Age			
18–34 years	799	39.46	1.97
35–49 years	716	32.21	1.56
50–64 years	416	18.04	1.15
65 years or more	164	10.30	1.74
Education			
11 years or less	316	15.15	1.50
12 years	371	17.64	1.16
13–16 years	1018	47.04	2.20
17 years or more	389	20.17	1.93
Marital Status			
Married	1376	65.39	2.01
Never	512	25.05	1.53
Widowed/Separated/Divorced	205	9.56	1.02
Employment			
Employed	1383	63.83	1.58
Out of labor force/Others	565	29.80	1.69
Unemployed	145	6.38	0.63
Income			
$0–14,999	815	42.55	1.24
$15,000–34,999	446	25.22	1.37
$35,000–74,999	475	23.96	0.99
$75,000+	172	8.27	1.00
Past 12-month Use of Services			
Generalist	85	4.25	0.50
Specialist	72	3.09	0.47
Social Support			
Family or relative support	2086	10.91	0.12
Friend support	2087	10.67	0.11
Family harmony	2089	6.11	0.04
Friend harmony	2088	6.64	0.03

Variations by US-Born Asian Subgroups: Use of Generalist Services

Friend support, marital status, and *work status* was strongly associated with use of generalist services for US-born Chinese. The odds of using generalist services among US-born Chinese decreased by 24% when friend support increased by one score (OR $=$ 0.76, p $=$ 0.043). *Family support* and *work status* was strongly associated with using generalist services for US-born Other Asian. For Other Asians, the odds of using generalist services increased nearly threefold when family support increased by one score (OR $=$ 2.98, p $=$ 0.021). *Friend harmony* and *marital status* were strong predictors for using generalist services for US-born Chinese. The odds of using generalist services among US-born Chinese increased threefold when friend harmony increased by one score (OR $=$ 3.08, p $=$ 0.006) (Table 2).

Variations by US-Born Asian Subgroups: Use of Specialist Services

For US-born Other Asian, *family support*, *family harmony*, *friend harmony*, and *martial status* were strongly associated with using specialist services. The odds of using specialist services among US-born Other Asian increased two and a halffold (OR $=$ 2.48, p $=$ 0.000) and about fourfold (OR $=$ 4.20, p $=$ 0.001) when family support and friend harmony increased by one score, respectively. But the odds of using specialist services decreased by 54% when family harmony increased by one score (OR $=$ 0.44, p $=$ 0.026) (Table 3).

Variations by Foreign-Born Asian Subgroups: Use of Generalist and Specialist Services

Friend support and *work status* was strongly associated with use of generalist services for foreign-born Filipinos. The odds of using generalist services among foreign-born Filipinos increased by 27% when friend support increased by one score (OR $=$ 1.27, p $=$ 0.055). *Friend harmony* and *marital status* was strongly associated with use of specialist services for foreign-born Chinese. The odds of using specialist services for foreign-born Chinese increased about twofold when friend harmony increased by one score (OR $=$ 2.07, p $=$ 0.057) (Table 4).

Social Support and Use of Generalist Services

Because primary care providers are typically the first point of contact for individuals seeking health care services, our model analyzed the use of generalist services. Interestingly, reliance on *family support* and *friend support* was not strongly associated with use of generalist services (Table 5). *Family harmony, nativity, employment status,* and *income* were significant predictors for using generalist services. Our results indicate that the odds of

Table 2. Logistic Regression Model for Social Support and Use of Generalist Services for US-Born Asians.

	US-Born Chinese $N = 125$			US-Born Other Asian $N = 152$			US-Born Chinese $N = 125$		
	Beta coeff.	p-value	OR (95% CI)	Beta coeff.	p-value	OR (95% CI)	Beta coeff.	p-value	OR (95% CI)
Social Support									
Family support	-0.46	0.150	0.63 (0.33, 1.19)	1.09	0.021*	2.98 (1.19, 7.49)			
Friend support	-0.28	0.043*	0.76 (0.58, 0.99)	-0.40	0.157	0.67 (0.38, 1.18)			
Family harmony							-0.27	0.429	0.76 (0.38, 1.52)
Friend harmony							1.13	0.006**	3.08 (1.39, 6.82)
Sex									
Male[†]									
Female	0.78	0.066	2.19 (0.95, 5.07)	0.47	0.530	1.61 (0.35, 7.37)	0.69	0.157	1.99 (0.75, 5.27)
Marital Status									
Married[†]									
Single	-0.29	0.814	0.75 (0.06, 8.96)	-1.62	0.075	0.20 (0.03, 1.19)	-0.71	0.241	0.49 (0.14, 1.66)
Widowed/Separated/ Divorced	3.02	0.040*	20.54 (1.16, 364.27)	2.79	0.143	16.27 (0.37, 720.44)	2.13	0.010**	8.42 (1.69, 41.98)
Work Status									
Employed[†]									
Out of labor force	-0.27	0.837	0.76 (0.05, 10.94)	1.13	0.595	3.09 (0.04, 224.88)	-0.42	0.785	0.66 (0.03, 14.91)
Unemployed	-4.26	0.047*	0.01 (0.00, 0.96)	6.45	0.005**	629.93 (7.30, 54365.52)	-3.23	0.120	0.04 (0.00, 2.45)
K10 Psychological Distress	0.56	0.000***	1.76 (1.32, 2.34)	0.56	0.045*	1.74 (1.01, 3.00)	0.47	0.000***	1.61 (1.23, 2.09)

[†] Reference category, * $p \leqslant .05$, ** $p \leqslant .01$, *** $p \leqslant .001$.

Table 3. Logistic Regression Model for Social Support and Use of Specialist Services for US-Born Asians.

	US-Born Other Asian ($N = 152$)			US-Born Other Asian ($N = 152$)		
	Beta coeff.	p-value	OR (95% CI)	Beta coeff.	p-value	OR (95% CI)
Social Support						
Family support	0.91	0.000***	2.48 (1.52, 4.07)			
Friend support	−0.24	0.271	0.78 (0.50, 1.22)			
Family harmony				−0.82	0.026*	0.44 (0.22, 0.90)
Friend harmony				1.44	0.001***	4.20 (1.77, 9.96)
Sex						
Male†						
Female	−0.25	0.800	0.78 (0.10, 5.84)	−0.40	0.711	0.67 (0.07, 6.08)
Marital Status						
Married†						
Single	−0.28	0.869	0.76 (0.03, 22.45)	0.52	0.768	1.69 (0.05, 61.32)
Widowed/Separated/ Divorced	2.10	0.005**	8.20 (1.95, 34.53)	2.70	0.002**	14.88 (2.69, 82.33)
Work Status						
Employed†						
Out of labor force	0.21	0.844	1.23 (0.15, 10.39)	1.47	0.299	4.33 (0.26, 73.34)
Unemployed						
K10 Psychological Distress	0.31	0.024*	1.36 (1.04, 1.78)	0.10	0.173	1.11 (0.95, 1.29)

† Reference category, * $p \leqslant .05$, ** $p \leqslant .01$, *** $p \leqslant .001$.

using generalist services among total sample decreased by 24% when family harmony increased by one score (OR = 0.76, p = 0.036). Compared to US-born Asians, foreign-born Asian were less likely to use generalist services (OR = 0.43, CI 0.19, 0.97). Individuals out of the labor force (OR = 5.63, CI 2.54, 12.50) and those who were unemployed (OR = 5.65, CI 1.73, 18.47) were five and a half times more likely to use generalist services compared to those who were employed (Table 6).

Social Support and Use of Specialist Services

Similarly, *family support* and *friend support* were not significant predictors for use of specialty mental health care services (Table 7). *Friend harmony*, *gender*, *marital status*, and *income* were significant predictors for using specialty mental health care services (Table 8). Our results on the use of specialist services do not support our hypothesis. Rather, the odds of using specialty mental health care services increased about two-thirds (or 63%) when friend

Table 4. Logistic Regression Model for Social Support and Use of Services for Foreign-Born Asians.

	Foreign-Born Filipinos ($N = 349$)			Foreign-Born Chinese ($N = 473$)		
	Generalist services			Specialist services		
	Beta coeff.	*p*-value	OR (95% CI)	Beta coeff.	*p*-value	OR (95% CI)
Social Support						
Family support	−0.02	0.890	0.98 (0.77, 1.26)			
Friend support	0.24	0.055*	1.27 (0.99, 1.62)			
Family harmony				0.09	0.754	1.09 (0.61, 1.96)
Friend harmony				0.73	0.057*	2.07 (0.98, 4.41)
Sex						
Male†						
Female	0.67	0.326	1.96 (0.50, 7.69)	−0.85	0.239	0.43 (0.10, 1.81)
Marital Status						
Married†						
Single	−0.50	0.502	0.60 (0.13, 2.75)	2.22	0.000***	9.24 (3.21, 26.56)
Widowed/Separated/ Divorced	0.16	0.809	1.18 (0.30, 4.57)	0.50	0.565	1.64 (0.29, 9.40)
Work Status						
Employed†						
Out of labor force	1.65	0.025*	5.23 (1.24, 22.09)	−0.73	0.310	0.48 (0.11, 2.05)
Unemployed	–	–	–	–	–	–
K10 Psychological Distress	0.10	0.066	1.11 (0.99, 1.24)	0.08	0.101	1.08 (0.98, 1.18)

† Reference category, * $p \leqslant .05$, *** $p \leqslant .001$.

harmony increased by one score (OR = 1.63, p = 0.002). Compared to men, women were less likely to use specialist services (OR = 0.39, CI 0.18, 0.88). Those who were widowed, separated, or divorced were five times more likely to use specialist services (OR = 5.29, CI 2.65, 10.55) compared to married individuals. Those with incomes over $75,000 were nearly six times more likely to use specialist services (OR = 5.93, CI 1.95, 18.02) than those who earned $14,999 or less.

DISCUSSION

Our study results aimed to measure whether levels of social support facilitated the use of mental health services among Asian American adults. Some of our findings are noteworthy. Our partial analyses of Asian subgroups indicated variations in the use of general medical care and specialty mental health care among Vietnamese, Filipino, Chinese, and

Table 5. Logistic Regression Model for Social Support and Use of Generalist Services.

	Generalist ($N = 1898$)		
	Beta coeff.	p-value	OR (95% CI)
Social Support			
Family support	0.09	0.087	1.09 (0.99, 1.21)
Friend support	0.10	0.293	1.10 (0.92, 1.32)
Gender			
Male[†]			
Female	−0.08	0.761	0.92 (0.55, 1.56)
Nativity			
U.S.-born[†]			
Foreign-born	−0.72	0.109	0.49 (0.20, 1.19)
Age			
18–34 years[†]			
35–49 years	0.31	0.483	1.36 (0.56, 3.31)
50–64 years	0.51	0.359	1.67 (0.54, 5.10)
65 years or more	0.73	0.157	2.07 (0.74, 5.77)
Education			
11 years or less[†]			
12 years	−0.73	0.231	0.48 (0.14, 1.63)
13–16 years	−0.30	0.447	0.74 (0.33, 1.64)
17 years or more	−1.16	0.059	0.31 (0.09, 1.05)
Marital Status			
Married[†]			
Single	−0.26	0.626	0.77 (0.27, 2.23)
Widowed/Separated/Divorced	0.50	0.168	1.65 (0.80, 3.38)
Employment			
Employed[†]			
Out of labor force	1.64	0.000***	5.14 (2.29, 11.56)
Unemployed	1.63	0.005**	5.10 (1.66, 15.69)
Income			
0–14,999[†]			
15,000–34,999	0.96	0.010**	2.61 (1.27, 5.34)
35,000–74,999	0.65	0.249	1.91 (0.62, 5.91)
75,000+	0.49	0.549	1.63 (0.31, 8.53)
K10 Psychological Distress	0.16	0.000***	1.17 (1.11, 1.23)

[†]Reference category, **$p \leqslant .01$, *** $p \leqslant .001$.

Other Asian groups. Variations were mediated by nativity. In other words, US-born and foreign-born Asian subgroups used generalist and specialist services in varying degrees. The association of nativity with social support also revealed interesting results. While family support and friend harmony

Table 6. Logistic Regression Model for Social Support and Use of Generalist Services.

	Generalist ($N = 1,899$)		
	Beta coeff.	p-value	OR (95% CI)
Social Support			
Family harmony	−0.27	0.036*	0.76 (0.59, 0.98)
Friend harmony	0.18	0.260	1.20 (0.87, 1.66)
Gender			
Male[†]			
Female	−0.08	0.777	0.92 (0.51, 1.67)
Nativity			
US-born[†]			
Foreign-born	−0.84	0.043*	0.43 (0.19, 0.97)
Age			
18–34 years[†]			
35–49 years	0.17	0.701	1.18 (0.49, 2.87)
50–64 years	0.45	0.392	1.56 (0.55, 4.46)
65 years or more	0.44	0.339	1.56 (0.61, 3.95)
Education			
11 years or less[†]			
12 years	−0.64	0.279	0.53 (0.16, 1.73)
13–16 years	−0.26	0.498	0.77 (0.36, 1.66)
17 years or more	−1.00	0.082	0.37 (0.12, 1.15)
Marital Status			
Married[†]			
Never	−0.18	0.742	0.84 (0.28, 2.48)
Widowed/Separated/Divorced	0.46	0.159	1.58 (0.83, 3.01)
Employment			
Employed[†]			
Out of labor force	1.73	0.000***	5.63 (2.54, 12.50)
Unemployed	1.73	0.005**	5.65 (1.73, 18.47)
Income			
$0–14,999[†]			
$15,000–34,999	1.06	0.005**	2.90 (1.40, 5.99)
$35,00074,999	0.77	0.188	2.16 (0.67, 6.91)
$75,000+	0.71	0.408	2.04 (0.36, 11.55)
K10 Psychological Distress	0.14	0.000***	1.15 (1.10, 1.21)

[†] Reference category, * $p \leqslant .05$, ** $p \leqslant .01$, *** $p \leqslant .001$.

increased the odds of using specialist services, family harmony decreased the odds of using specialty mental health care services.

In our regression models (Tables 5 through 8), we found that *types of social support* (family and friend support versus family and friend harmony)

Table 7. Logistic Regression Model for Social Support and Use of Specialist Services.

	Specialist ($N = 1,901$)		
	Beta coeff.	p-value	OR (95% CI)
Social Support			
Family support	0.10	0.163	1.11 (0.96, 1.28)
Friend support	−0.03	0.783	0.97 (0.79, 1.19)
Gender			
Male[†]			
Female	0.26	0.408	1.29 (0.69, 2.41)
Nativity			
U.S.-born[†]			
Foreign-born	−0.94	0.025*	0.39 (0.17, 0.89)
Age			
18–34 years[†]			
35–49 years	−0.06	0.905	0.94 (0.33, 2.70)
50–64 years	0.72	0.155	2.06 (0.75, 5.64)
65 years or more	−0.45	0.564	0.64 (0.13, 3.09)
Education			
11 years or less[†]			
12 years	0.43	0.432	1.54 (0.51, 4.63)
13–16 years	0.63	0.233	1.87 (0.66, 5.32)
17 years or more	−0.03	0.969	0.98 (0.26, 3.62)
Marital Status			
Married[†]			
Single	0.64	0.169	1.89 (0.75, 4.76)
Widowed/Separated/Divorced	1.64	0.000***	5.15 (2.47, 10.75)
Employment			
Employed[†]			
Out of labor force	0.63	0.090	1.87 (0.90, 3.87)
Unemployed	0.12	0.724	1.13 (0.56, 2.31)
Income			
0–14,999[†]			
15,000–34,999	−0.30	0.564	0.74 (0.26, 2.10)
35,000–74,999	0.16	0.723	1.17 (0.48, 2.85)
75,000+	1.46	0.012*	4.31 (1.40, 13.29)
K10 Psychological Distress	0.15	0.000***	1.16 (1.11, 1.21)

[†] Reference category, * $p \leqslant .05$, *** $p \leqslant .001$.

influenced the use of mental health services. Results showing that *friend harmony* leads to the use of specialist services could be partly explained by the instrumental aid provided by friends. In other words, individuals could be receiving advice and information from friends on availability of mental

Table 8. Logistic Regression Model for Social Support and Use of Specialist Services.

	Specialist ($N = 1,902$)		
	Beta coeff.	p-value	OR (95% CI)
Social Support			
Family harmony	−0.25	0.143	0.78 (0.55, 1.09)
Friend harmony	0.49	0.002**	1.63 (1.20, 2.22)
Gender			
Male[†]			
Female	−0.93	0.024*	0.39 (0.18, 0.88)
Nativity			
US-born[†]			
Foreign-born	0.18	0.534	1.19 (0.67, 2.11)
Age			
18–34 years[†]			
35–49 years	−0.04	0.934	0.96 (0.37, 2.53)
50–64 years	0.84	0.063	2.31 (0.95, 5.60)
65 years or more	−0.50	0.484	0.61 (0.15, 2.53)
Education			
11 years or less[†]			
12 years	0.43	0.425	1.53 (0.52, 4.50)
13–16 years	0.57	0.244	1.77 (0.66, 4.75)
17 years or more	0.08	0.891	1.09 (0.31, 3.83)
Marital Status			
Married[†]			
Never	0.75	0.157	2.13 (0.74, 6.14)
Widowed/Separated/Divorced	1.67	0.000***	5.29 (2.65, 10.55)
Employment			
Employed[†]			
Out of labor force	0.69	0.059	2.00 (0.97, 4.13)
Unemployed	0.06	0.883	1.06 (0.48, 2.33)
Income			
$0–14,999[†]			
$15,000–34,999	−0.20	0.709	0.82 (0.28, 2.43)
$35,000–74,999	0.21	0.635	1.24 (0.50, 3.04)
$75,000+	1.78	0.002**	5.93 (1.95, 18.02)
K10 Psychological Distress	0.14	0.000***	1.15 (1.10, 1.20)

[†] Reference category, * $p \leqslant .05$, ** $p \leqslant .01$, *** $p \leqslant .001$.

health services. *Friend harmony* appears more significant than family harmony perhaps because individuals feel less distress, less demands, and fewer expectations from friends compared to family. Norms that dictate friend versus family relationships may differ (Turner, Pearlin, & Mullan, 1998).

Analyses with all four scales (family support, friend support, family harmony, and friend harmony) were not significant (data not shown). We also analyzed social variables such as *family pride*, *family cohesion*, and *family conflict*. Our analyses revealed that including these variables with our social support variables did not result in significant findings (data not shown). Family pride, family cohesion, and family conflict were not strong predictors of using mental health services.

CONCLUSIONS

Some limitations of our study must be noted. Our partial analyses of Asian subgroups may limit detection of significant differences among Vietnamese, Filipino, Chinese, and Other Asian because of our limited sample sizes for each group. Another limitation is the exclusion of other variables such as acculturation, discrimination, generational differences, and years living in the US, which may explain differences of service use.

Despite our limitations, our study has important implications for providing mental health care to Asian Americans. Specifically, further research is necessary to explain between-group differences and within-group differences (e.g., US-born versus foreign-born Filipinos). Further research requires inclusion of additional factors to determine the overall low utilization of mental health services by Asian Americans. Various measures of *acculturation*, defined as the "process of adaptation to cultural values, behavior, knowledge, and identity of the dominant society" (Kim & Omizo, 2003), may not fully capture reasons for use and non-use of mental health services. Conflicting evidence exists on whether levels of acculturation and the attitudes and willingness of Asian Americans influence seeking professional psychological services. The role of acculturation and understanding health is complex and may differ across various ethnic groups (Dey & Lucas, 2006), especially when taking into account differences in migration histories (Kuo & Porter, 1998) and stressors related to acculturation (Takeuchi, Mokuau, & Chun, 1992). Utilization of formal health care services is influenced by social, cultural, and economic contexts (LeClere, Jensen, & Biddlecom, 1994). For Asian Americans, immigration-related factors were associated with mental disorders, but in different ways for men and women. Future studies will need to examine gender as an important factor in specifying the association between immigration and mental health (Takeuchi et al., 2007).

In addition to measuring acculturative stress, discrimination and racism could also serve as indicators of stressful life events and experiences which could lead to use of mental health services. The research on the impact of racism on Asian Americans is lacking (Alvarez & Kimura, 2001). Other factors to consider in examining utilization of mental health care services by Asian Americans are the availability of services, access to services, and severity (degree) of mental illness. Additional social factors also need to be explored to determine if acculturation, discrimination, and racism contribute to or inhibit use of mental health services. Identifying the specific social factors that influence the use of or inhibit the use of mental health services can contribute to providing culturally competent care. If general medical care providers can better recognize depressive symptoms, for example, primary care physicians can serve as the pathway to mental health referrals or treatment (Chung et al., 2003).

ACKNOWLEDGMENTS

The NLAAS was supported by U01 MH62209 and U01 MH62207 from the National Institute of Mental Health and by the Office of Behavioral and Social Science Research and the Substance Abuse and Mental Health Services Administration. Dr. Nicdao was supported by T32 MH067555 from the National Institute of Mental Health and by University of Michigan, NIMH Racial, Ethnic, and Cultural Disparities in Mental Health Training Program.

REFERENCES

Abe-Kim, J., Takeuchi, D. T., Hong, S., Zane, N., Sue, S., Spencer, M., Appel, H., Nicdao, E., & Alegria, M. (2007). Use of mental health-related services among immigrant and US-born Asian Americans: Results from the national Latino and Asian American study. *American Journal of Public Health, 97*(1), 91–98.

Alvarez, A. N., & Kimura, E. F. (2001). Asian Americans and racial identity: Dealing with racism and snowballs. *Journal of Mental Health Counseling, 23*(3), 192–206.

Barreto, R. M., & Segal, S. P. (2005). Use of mental health services by Asian Americans. *Psychiatric Services, 56*(6), 746–748.

Chung, H., Teresi, J., Guarnaccia, P., Meyers, B., Holmes, D., Bobrowitz, T., Eimicke, J., & Ferran, E., Jr. (2003). Depressive symptoms and psychiatric distress in low income Asian and Latino primary care patients: Prevalence and recognition. *Community Mental Health Journal, 39*(1), 33–46.

Cobb, S. (1976). Social support as a moderator of life stress. *Psychosomatic Medicine, 38*(5), 300–314.

Dey, A. N., & Lucas, J. W. (2006). Physical and mental health characteristics of U.S.- and foreign-born adults: United States, 1998–2003. Advance data from vital and health statistics (No. 369). Hyattsville, MD: National Center for Health Statistics.

Gellis, Z. D. (2003). Kin and nonkin social supports in a community sample of Vietnamese immigrants. *Social Work, 48*(2), 248.

Heeringa, S., Wagner, J., Torres, M., Duan, N., Adams, T., & Berglund, P. (2004). Sample designs and sampling methods for the collaborative psychiatric epidemiology studies (CPES). *International Journal of Methods in Psychiatric Research, 13*(4), 221–240.

Herrick, C. A., & Brown, H. N. (1998). Underutilization of mental health services by Asian-Americans residing in the United States. *Issues in Mental Health Nursing, 19*(3), 225–240.

Hu, T.-W., Snowden, L., Jerrell, J., & Nguyen, T. (1991). Ethnic populations in public mental health: Services choice and level of use. *American Journal of Public Health, 81*(11), 1429–1434.

Kaplan, B. H., Cassel, J. C., & Gore, S. (1977). Social support and health. *Medical Care, 15*(5(Suppl)), 47–58.

Kim, B. S. K., & Omizo, M. M. (2003). Asian cultural values, attitudes toward seeking professional psychological help, and willingness to see a counselor. *Counseling Psychologist, 31*(3), 343–361.

Kuo, J., & Porter, K. (1998). Health status of Asian Americans: United States, 1992–94. Advance data from vital and health statistics (No. 298). Hyattsville, MD: National Center for Health Statistics.

LeClere, F. B., Jensen, L., & Biddlecom, A. (1994). Health care utilization, family context, and adaptation among immigrants to the United States. *Journal of Health and Social Behavior, 35*(4), 370–384.

Lincoln, K. D., Chatters, L. M., & Taylor, R. J. (2005). Social support, traumatic events, and depressive symptoms among African Americans. *Journal of Marriage and Family, 67*(3), 754–766.

Mulvaney-Day, N. E., Alegria, M., & Sribney, W. (2007). Social cohesion, social support, and health among Latinos in the United States. *Social Science and Medicine, 64*, 477–495.

Okazaki, S. (2000). Treatment delay among Asian-American patients with severe mental illness. *American Journal of Orthopsychiatry, 70*(1), 58–64.

Takeuchi, D., Mokuau, N., & Chun, C. (1992). Mental health services for Asian Americans and Pacific Islanders. *Journal of Mental Health Administration, 19*(3), 237–245.

Takeuchi, D. T., & Kim, K. F. (2000). Enhancing mental health services delivery for diverse populations. *Contemporary Sociology, 29*(1), 74–83.

Takeuchi, D. T., Zane, N., Hong, S., Chae, D., Gong, F., Gee, G., Walton, E., Sue, S., & Alegria, M. (2007). Immigration-related factors and mental disorders among Asian Americans. *American Journal of Public Health, 97*(1), 84–90.

Taylor, S., Sherman, D., Kim, H. S., Jarcho, J., Takagi, K., & Dunagan, M. (2004). Culture and social support: Who seeks it and why? *Journal of Personality and Social Psychology, 87*(3), 354–362.

Thoits, P. A. (1982). Conceptual, methodological, and theoretical problems in studying social support as a buffer against life stress. *Journal of Health and Social Behavior, 23*(June), 145–159.

Thoits, P. A. (1984). Explaining distributions of psychological vulnerability: Lack of social support in the face of life stress. *Social Forces, 63*(2), 453–481.

Thoits, P. A. (1986). Social support as coping assistance. *Journal of Consulting and Clinical Psychology, 54*(4), 416–423.

Thoits, P. A. (1995). Stress, coping, and social support processes: Where are we? What next? *Journal of Health and Social Behavior, 35*(5), 53–79.

Turner, H. A., Pearlin, L. I., & Mullan, J. T. (1998). Sources and determinants of social support for caregivers of persons with AIDS. *Journal of Health and Social Behavior, 39*(2), 137–151.

Yamashiro, G., & Matsuoka, J. K. (1997). Help-seeking among Asian and Pacific Americans: A multiperspective analysis. *Social Work, 42*(2), 176–186.

SECTION 5:
BROADER CONSIDERATIONS ABOUT POPULATION HEALTH IN SPECIALIZED POPULATIONS AND ACROSS COUNTRIES

"FALLING THROUGH THE CRACKS": HEALTH CARE NEEDS OF THE OLDER HOMELESS POPULATION AND THEIR IMPLICATIONS ☆

Dennis P. Watson, Christine George and Christopher Walker

ABSTRACT

The homelessness of those 50–64, older homeless people, is a growing problem in the United States. This chapter seeks to understand the unique healthcare issues faced by this population. Data in the city of Chicago was collected and analyzed through a variety of qualitative and quantitative methods. Data included answers to survey questions by older homeless individuals, interviews with providers and older homeless individuals, focus

☆The data analyzed in this chapter is from a collaborative research project between Loyola University Chicago Center for Urban Research and Learning and the Chicago Alliance to End Homelessness that was supported by the Retirement Research Foundation.

Care for Major Health Problems and Population Health Concerns:
Impacts on Patients, Providers and Policy
Research in the Sociology of Health Care, Volume 26, 187–204
Copyright © 2008 by Emerald Group Publishing Limited
All rights of reproduction in any form reserved
ISSN: 0275-4959/doi:10.1016/S0275-4959(08)26009-6

groups with older homeless individuals, and agency data from homeless service organizations. Findings agree with previous research that shows a growth in the homeless population, the greater number and severity of health problems in the population, the significant number of barriers that the population encounters in obtaining health care, housing, and jobs, and the concern with preventative health that the older homeless have. After outlining these findings, this chapter offers policy and program recommendations for the larger health care and homeless service systems.

An emerging issue in the United States is the growth of homelessness among older adults, specifically those age 50–64 (hereafter known as the older homeless).[1] This population is important to look at separately from the homeless population in general because it faces unique problems related to aging and cohort effects. These problems have immediate implications for whether or not the needs of the older homeless are being adequately met/ addressed, as well as broader implications for the state of health care throughout the nation.

There are two important structural issues existing in the broader system that serves the homeless population, which need to be taken into consideration when looking at the older homeless. First, it should be recognized that the unique situations of the older homeless may interfere with their abilities to benefit from traditional services devised with the issues of the younger homeless in mind. Second, this population is not always eligible for public benefits that older individuals, those over 64, may easily qualify for. This can mean that many of this population may end up suffering with problems until they "age into services/benefits." Recognizing these structural issues, this chapter seeks to understand the demographic profile and needs that are unique the older homeless population. The information presented in this chapter has implications for all of the United States considering the expected rise in the number of older homeless individuals as the "baby boomer" generation ages (Cohen, 1999; Dietz & Wright, 2003) and recent studies showing the already large number of older homeless existing in some major metropolitan areas of the United States (Hahn, Kushel, Bangsberg, Riley, & Moss, 2005; North, Eyrich, Pollio, & Spitznagel, 2004; Smith, 2003). After describing some of the previous research looking at this population and its health concerns, this chapter discusses findings from a study in Chicago that used a mixed methods approach to better understand the health care issues of the older homeless population and provides a discussion of some of the larger implications seen by the researchers.

BACKGROUND ON AGING AND HOMELESSNESS

Brickner and Scanlan (1990) have suggested a need to pay more attention to the diversity and uniqueness of the homeless population. This is especially important for service providers because recognizing differences among subgroups of homeless individuals can lead to better assessment of the barriers their clients encounter and, consequently, a higher level of service. One such subgroup of homeless people who face unique barriers is the older homeless population. In order to understand the importance of this population and its relation to the larger health care system more adequately, it is necessary to identify what previous research has found regarding its current demographic trends and how health issues concerning homeless and housed older people differ, as well as how the health problems of the older homeless differ from the homeless population as a whole.

Trends in Aging and Homelessness

The older homeless make up a substantial portion of the general homeless population (Burt, Laudan, & Lee, 2001; Cohen, 1999; Rossi, 1989; Smith, 2003). Recently in Chicago and the surrounding suburbs, researchers for the Illinois Regional Roundtable on Homelessness (2002) found that 8.3% of homeless respondents in their sample were 55–64 years old (Smith, 2003). The Roundtable also conducted a survey of homeless service providers that places the figure of the older homeless at closer to 13.6% of the total homeless population (Smith, 2003). In addition to the significant number of older homeless in Chicago, other studies in large U.S. cities have pointed to the aging of the homeless population in recent years. For instance, a longitudinal study by North et al. (2004) found that the percentage of homeless between 45 and 64 had more than doubled between 1990 and 2000 in St. Louis. In San Francisco, the median age of the homeless increased 9 years from 1990 to 2003; one-third of the homeless population were aged 50 and older. In addition to observed growth, Cohen (1999), one of the most recognized researchers on the homelessness of older people, has predicted a doubling of the older homeless population on the national level within 30 years.

Health and Health Care of Older Homeless Persons

It has consistently been shown that homeless individuals are at greater risk for certain health problems than people who are housed (Dennis, Levine, &

Osher, 1991; Dickey, Normand, Weiss, Drake, & Azenie, 2002; Gelberg, Andersen, & Leake, 2002; Resenbaum & Zuvekas, 1995; Scharer, Berson, & Brickner, 1990). In conjunction with this risk, it has also been shown that homeless individuals are not utilizing services for their health problems despite high levels of need within the population (Padgett, Struening, & Andrews, 1990), and that the lack of available services for this population has resulted in the underutilization of preventative and primary health care and the overutilization of emergency room services (Han, Wells, & Taylor, 2003; Sachs-Ericsson, Wise, Debrody, & Paniucki, 1999). Taking this into consideration with the number of health-related problems associated with aging, it is reasonable to assume that older homeless individuals have a greater number and more chronic/complicated health problems than younger homeless, and this has been confirmed by previous studies (Cohen & Skolovsky, 1989; Cohen, Teresi, & Holmes, 1988; Crane & Warnes, 2001; Gelberg, Linn, & Mayer-Oakes, 1990).

In studies from both the United States and United Kingdom, health problems related to aging were shown to be greater in the older homeless population than in those in the same age group who are housed (Cohen & Skolovsky, 1989; Crane & Warnes, 2001; Gelberg et al., 1990). Additionally, research specific to the United States has shown that a large portion of the older homeless are lacking benefits which could help them obtain medical services (Hatchett, 2004; Kushel, Vittinghoff, & Hass, 2001; Smith, 2003). Despite this greater need, the homeless service system has often been pointed to as wrongly conceptualizing or ignoring health issues related to aging (Crane & Warnes, 2005; Hecht & Coyle, 2001). For instance, one study showed that while medical problems such as arthritis, hypertension, diabetes, and pneumonia can cause older homeless persons to receive some attention from service providers, the seriousness of these health issues are often overlooked (Kutza & Keigher, 1991). In an attempt to address this issue, researchers have advocated for more thorough health screenings or medical assessments when older homeless individuals interact with service providers in hopes that this will set the course for long-term intervention (Kutza & Keigher, 1991).

Other research has shown that homeless people are willing to obtain care if they feel it is important (Gelberg et al., 2002) and if it is accessible (Kushel et al., 2001), but there is a lack of fit between the needs of the homeless and the organization of health services (Gallagher, Andersen, Kogel & Gelberg, 1997) that makes access to preventative care difficult. While it is easy to see the effect lack of preventative and regular primary care for acute or chronic conditions may have on older homeless individuals themselves (i.e., worsening of problems, more complications, higher mortality), the effect that lack of treatment has on the nation is also important. Emergency room visits and acute care are two examples of how the cost of care for those with severe heath problems and no access to services affect the broader healthcare system, as well as the broader economy. Emergency and acute care services cost more than regular and preventative care. The cost for these more expensive services is shouldered by the U.S. government when hospitals do not get paid for them, and this burden is often times not covered completely by the federal budget. For instance, the price of uncompensated care was estimated at 41 billion dollars in 2004, but the U.S. government had only projected enough funds to pay for 85% of this total cost (Kaiser Family Foundation, 2007). Additionally, hospitals have been estimated to pay about 34 billion dollars a year on uncompensated care that is often provided for preventable diseases or those that could be treated more easily with an earlier diagnosis (Institute of Medicine, 2003), and this puts financial strain on hospitals' ability to provide higher level care for non-acute conditions (The Commonwealth Fund, 2003).

The findings of past research on the growth of the older homeless population and their greater health care needs in combination with the financial strain that uncompensated care has on the larger U.S. health care system and economy illuminates the need for understanding health care problems and barriers to services that are particular to the older homeless. If research is able to provide answers to some of the questions that surround this population and their health care needs, then service providers may find less costly ways to address their problems, which would have positive benefits for the health care system as a whole.

METHODS

Data collected for this study were from five different sources (Table 1); (1) archival data from a representative survey of homeless individuals in Cook County was used for statistical analysis, (2) interviews were conducted with service providers, (3) administrative data from homeless service agencies was requested, (4) and focus groups and (5) life history interviews were conducted with older homeless individuals.

Providers and homeless individuals were recruited from participating organizations identified with the help of the Chicago Alliance to End Homelessness. Participating agencies represented a wide variety of specialties in the provision of services to homeless individuals (i.e., shelter/housing, meals, and clinical services) to a wide variety of specific homeless populations.

Table 1.   Description of Data Sources, Methods of Collection, and
Analysis Techniques.

Data Source	Method	Analysis Techniques	N
Providers	Structured interviews	Quantitative analysis of close-ended questions and qualitative analysis of open-ended questions	56[a]
	Administrative data[b]	Quantitative analysis	23
Homeless men	Focus groups[c]	Qualitative analysis	8
and women	Life history interviews[c]	Qualitative analysis	10
	Archival data[b]	Quantitative analysis	123

[a]This number is higher than the total number of participating organizations for interviews because we conducted two interviews with one agency at two different locations.
[b]Primary quantitative analysis conducted by Marilyn Krogh, PhD, Loyola University Chicago.
[c]Focus groups and Interviews conducted by Judith Wittner, PhD, Loyola University Chicago.

Archival Data

Quantitative analysis relied on standard statistical techniques, such as means and cross-tabulations, used to examine the demographics of this population, their distinct patterns/paths of homelessness, and their service needs. Data from the Illinois Regional Roundtable (2002) was provided to the research team for analysis by the University of Illinois, Chicago. The demographics of the population are shown in Table 2.

Administrative Data

To get a more up-to-date picture of the trends in the older homeless population, this report also synthesizes administrative data collected over the past 5 years from participating agencies. About half of the service providers in the sample kept individual level demographic records about their clients, some for all 5 past years, some for 3 years, and some just for the current year. While these records are not complete, they provide the best available snapshot of recent trends.

Provider Interviews

Fifty-five agencies agreed to participate in provider interviews. The interview script was designed to collect the following data: (1) population

Table 2. Demographic Profile of All Clients Aged 50–64 Living in Chicago in 2001.

Variable	Aged 50–64 (%)	Variable	Aged 50–64 (%)
Male	76	Currently married	5
Black	63	Has children <18 yrs old	20
Institutional/foster care during childhood	10	Working full-time	11
Non-parental relative care in childhood	17	Working part-time, day labor, or other	18
High school graduate	59	Not working	37
Active duty veteran	18	Retired/disabled	29
Ever incarcerated	20	Never homeless	13
			$(N = 123)$

Table 3. Gender, Race, and Age of Focus Group Participants.

Gender	Male	Female			
	16	37			
Race	Black	White	Hispanic	Asian	
	48	3	1	1	
Age	50–54[a]	55–59	60–64	Unknown	
	34	15	3	1	$N = 53$

[a]One individual states she is actually 47, but represents herself as 50 because she was arrested and processed with identification that stated she was 50, an identification which she continues to use.

demographic data, (2) providers' observations of trends regarding the number of older homeless clients served, (3) the needs of the targeted population (4) any observed service gaps in the homeless system, (5) the providers' perception of the organizations capacity to serve the population, and (6) any policy-related issues/concerns.

Focus Groups and Interviews with Older Homeless Men and Women

Data were collected from eight focus groups of 5–12 homeless or formerly homeless men and women and in-depth life history interviews conducted with 10 homeless and formerly homeless individuals. The demographic profiles of the focus group and interview participants are presented in Table 3 and Table 4.

Table 4. Gender, Race, and Age of Life History Interview Participants.

Gender	Male	Female		
	5	5		
Race	Black	White	Hispanic	
	6	3	1	
Age	50–54	55–59	60–64	
	5	5	0	$N = 10$

Both focus groups and interviews were audio-recorded. Participants received a stipend of $30 for their participation.

FINDINGS

The Population is Growing

Most of the 55 agencies interviewed that serve homeless adults report seeing an increase in the population over the age of 50, and analysis of the administrative data support this, showing an average 11% yearly increase in this group for 22 agencies which there was more than 1 year of data for. According to the client service data from a convenience sample of 23 agencies, the percentage of clients aged 50 and over has been stable or growing from 2001 to 2006. Although some agencies had complete records back to 2001, and others only had more recent data, the trend is consistent for each group of agencies and for the set of agencies as a whole. Table 5 shows the total number and percentage of clients reported by the 23 agencies in selected years from 2001 to 2006.

As more agency data are available from 2001 to 2006, the number of clients reported increases from 1,825 to 21,635 (see Table 5). More significantly, however, the percentage of all the clients who are 50 years old and older increases from 19% to 24% (see Table 5). A variety of agencies reported data for different years, so this data must be interpreted with caution. However, it is likely that the percentage of older clients in these agencies service population is at least stable, and most likely growing.

Health Issues of the Older Homeless

Overall, the data show that a majority of the older homeless "fall through the cracks" in a system designed for either younger or older individuals.

Table 5. Total Number of Clients Reported by 23 Agencies and Percentage 50–64 for Selected Years[a].

	2001		2003		2005		2006	
Nine agencies	1,825	19%	1,642	23%	1,691	26%	1,446	29%
Five agencies			9,177	24%	12,806	24%	13,747	23%
Three agencies					3,044	12%	2,647	13%
Six agencies							3,795	29%
Total	1,825	19%	10,819	24%	17,541	22%	21,635	24%

[a]Due to the majority of these agencies record keeping protocols, all but six were able to provide numbers strictly for 50–64 year olds, however, considering what previous research has shown, it is unlikely that there are a large number of homeless over the age of 64 skewing the data. Six agencies reported data only on clients aged 50–64, so the percentages in the table are lower than they would be if all agencies reported on all clients aged 50 and over.

For instance, younger individuals who do not have health problems that are as pronounced may benefit from employment services, which can aid them in finding incomes through jobs that can help them to address their health problems, while individuals over 64 are more likely to be accepted for programs such as SSI, SSDI, and Medicare.

Chronic and Complicated Conditions
A quarter of the older homeless interviewed in the Roundtable study reported that they needed assistance obtaining medical services in the last 12 months, but only 66% of this group were able to obtain these services (Table 6).

Interview data shows that the older homeless are suffering from more and greater physical health problems than homeless who are younger. Providers reported that many older homeless have chronic and complicated health issues. Specifically, providers reported they see more problems of arthritis, vision, high blood pressure, age onset cancers, and diabetes in this population than younger ones.

> More chronic medical problems [are in the older homeless] than those younger ... [like] hypertension [and] diabetes developed through poor nutrition. Some medications can exasperate these problems, living on the streets, being poor, no follow up with medical care, higher risk for TB ... poor diet. (Provider)

It was also reported by providers that older homeless who have been exposed to certain medications (AIDS and psychotropic medications) for a number of years have health problems related to use of their prescriptions. For instance, individuals on anti-psychotic and HIV/AIDS medications for

Table 6.   Needed and Received Assistance in Last 12 Months for Physical
Health-Related Issues of Roundtable Respondents Aged 50–64.

Type of Assistance	Needed Assistance	Received Assistance
Vision	39	39
Dental care	37	18
Medication	33	66
Medical services	26	66
Nutrition	38	93
		$(N = 144)$

prolonged periods were reported to be more likely to suffer from metabolic
complications than those who have not been on them for as long.

Access to Health Care Services
Regardless of the high need for treatment of chronic and complicated health
problems, a number of providers pointed to insufficient access to the wide
range of specialists needed to serve this aging population, ranging from
dentists, and optometrists/optomologists to gerontologists, cardiologists,
rheumatologists, urologists, gastroenterologists. Due to these issues,
providers recognized a need for more healthcare screening of chronic
illnesses and age-related diseases than there has traditionally been. In
addition to this, consumers had experienced decreasing services and access
with the recent cutbacks at clinics and pharmacies in the area.

> Until recently … they were okay with health care, because their clients would go
> over to [the county hospital], but because of changes there is more difficulty, because
> they won't see them without documentation, and the satellite facilities used to be able
> to not charge them, but now there is a ten or fifteen dollar co-pay, which his clients
> cannot pay, so then they have to go to [the county hospital] and sit and wait long hours.
> (Provider)

As shown in the passage above, providers and consumers reported that
the increased difficulty of accessing services has led homeless individuals to
delay or skip seeking services for chronic conditions.

Connected to the lack of outpatient services, providers working in
housing programs also reported that some of their clients enter nursing
homes because there are not enough home health services or supportive
services programs that included home health care options.

Medication
In the 2001 survey, one-third of those who needed medication to manage their health problems were unable to get help in obtaining it (see Table 6). Reflecting this problem, providers and consumers often identified access of medication for the treatment of health problems as a large issue. The providers recognized that greater health needs come with a greater need for medication, and that older homeless, especially those recently released from prison, have a hard time obtaining prescriptions outside of free samples given by physicians, which run out quickly, hence, having only minor, if any, positive effects.

Dental and Vision
Many providers highlighted the dental and vision needs of the older homeless, as well as the inadequate system for addressing these problems.

> Dental care is also important and when their agency finds providers who will work with them to help this population, the providers typically become saturated due to the demand. (Provider)

In the Roundtable Study, over one-third of the older respondents reported a need for assistance in obtaining eye care/exams within the last year, but less than half (39%) were able to obtain any vision assistance (see Table 6). Dental care was an even worse scenario, with only a small fraction (18%) of those reporting a need for assistance in getting dental care within the last year receiving it (see Table 6).

Nutrition and Exercise
Thirty-eight percent of the individuals surveyed in the 2001 Roundtable study stated a need for assistance with obtaining food in the previous year. While most (see Table 6) of these individuals reported accessing food assistance, qualitative data collected from consumers and providers indicated that there were issues about regularity of meals and food quality in the homeless system.

When the issue of nutrition was brought up, it was commonly connected to health outcomes by both providers and consumers. For instance, in focus groups, individuals on medication described the problems associated with erratic meal schedules and taking medication.

> The biggest problem ... you're supposed to have three meals a day. Now, you're over 50, you don't have three meals a day. Now you're out there, you're trying to take medication if you get one meal a day. And then ... hypertension starts kicking in, diabetes, that's our biggest threat. That's mine. That's the biggest problem when you're

over 50. Thirty-year-old man, you know, he could get over it once he gets on his feet and gets a job. Over 50, getting medication like you're eating three meals a day, so it's dietary ... and the medication that you take once you get over 50, will all rush you into diabetes ... I'm not even talking about psych medication. That makes it even worse. (Focus group participant)

Focus group participants also reported that food preparation practices in many institutions that serve the homeless have not "caught up" with healthy cooking practices. This problem was also brought up by providers, and was connected to lack of healthy ingredients rather than dietary programming specific to the agency.

Getting nutritious food is a problem – fruits and vegetables – food pantry food is not fresh – they try to get produce but still a problem – the city has a food rescue program once a month that they use, but is meager. [we are] [t]rying to learn more about cooking and have the ... cooking be better. (Provider)

Another issue raised by focus group participants that is related to poor health outcomes is individuals' limited opportunities for healthy exercise. Some focus group participants made a connection between their lack of exercise and present and/or as yet undeveloped health problems.

I would like to see that 50 to 64 group talked to for some programs, such as like, the mayor has a program for seniors, like you can work out and stuff. And I used to sneak in those centers. But, you know, I'm not *old* old, but I would like to continue to be physically fit ... And so, uh, you know, to uh, prevent a lot of sickness and disease. But most of those programs are for 65 and over. Help me to stay strong while I am moving in that direction. (Focus group participant)

The above example also speaks to the lack of free public exercise programs, frequently identified as key to addressing health issues associated with aging are not as readily accessible to the younger "old" population as they are to those officially "seniors," 62.

Health Care Policy Barriers
Many aging homeless are not able to access Medicare and Medicaid. Providers who spoke on this issue pointed out how many homeless women over 50, who were covered by Medicaid have lost their status as their children "aged out" of system, and how many individual adults under 65, unless they are deemed disabled, are not eligible for Medicaid or Medicare. Individuals who had long histories of non-attachment to the labor force due to incarceration or other reasons also found themselves ineligible for Medicare.

Barriers Encountered Disability Benefits (SSI, SSDI)
The numerous reports by consumers and providers in Chicago of problems with Social Security Disability claims reflect a system-wide problem. Homeless individuals and providers reported their frustration with denials of applications and tying to understand and negotiate the benefit system.

> I went to the Social Security board and filled out the paperwork and went and seen the doctors and they told me I could get a job at McDonald's, Burger King, and I mean, I worked for the county for seventeen years … I broke my hip and that put me down … I go to the doctor now for therapy, I mean, I can't walk too far without my leg stiffening up on me, and so I talked to some lawyers and they told me to reapply all over again to Social Security. (Focus group participant)

> Trying to get somebody Social Security (SSI and SSDI) benefits is just a joke; it is time consuming and intense. [The] [r]ejection rate is around 88%. People start to get jaded … People just don't want to go through the process. (Provider)

Providers voiced frustration over not having staff trained to assist consumers in navigating the system. On the whole, agencies reported limited or no connections to legal advocates. Applications need documentation of physical and/or mental health problems. Obtaining this documentation for older individuals who have not had a consistent healthcare provider and whose records might be older records are hard to access and are not likely to be electronic. This issue is further compounded by individual's inability to pay for physicals needed in lieu of previous documentation.

DISCUSSION

The findings of this study support previous research that has looked at the issue of health care in the older homeless in a number of ways. First, all data collected point to the overwhelming need for health care services among the older homeless due to health problems and barriers that develop from the unique combination of issues related to both aging and homelessness. Second, discussions with providers regarding chronic and complicated health conditions of the older homeless support research that has pointed to the larger concentration of health problems of the older, in comparison to younger, homeless. Third, both the quantitative and qualitative data has shown that older homeless in Chicago, like those in other studies across the United States, face a number of barriers related to obtaining health care services; these barriers include lack of income and/or benefits, lack of an understanding of the health care needs of the older homeless, and a lack of medical providers willing to treat this population. Finally, discussions with older homeless men and women that centered on exercise and nutrition show that they are concerned with and willing to take preventative health measures, but accessing these services is challenging.

Ignoring the issues discussed above results in significant health care costs for the United States. When these problems go untreated, they can lead to even more costs for the public due to the need for more expensive treatments for this population. For instance, the chronic and complicated problems the older homeless face combined with difficulty accessing primary care services is a problem that can result in higher use of emergency room services for individuals. Another consequence that was not addressed adequately by the literature reviewed above is the concern providers in this study had with the large number of older homeless clients who end up in nursing homes due to the progression of their illness. Considering that nursing home care is around the clock and is many times indefinite, the costs to the general public may be even higher than emergency room use, and this needs to be considered in future research and when designing programs and policy.

Policy and Program Considerations

While difficult to overcome, there may be some strategies that can help to address these problems such as the building of partnerships between community service providers. Successful measures would ideally involve aging specialists and providers of other needed specialty services, for example, dentists, ophthamologists, and cardiologists. In order to be effective, efforts would need take a public health perspective and focus on early screening for medical problems and preventative care as much as servicing acute problems. In combination with screening, other preventative measures that should be a focus of programs are the provision of nutritious food, available means for exercise, and faster and more stable access to housing.

Many of the health care issues discussed above that the older homeless face are related to the lack of universal health care and non-family poverty targeted benefits for all ages. Navigation of the benefit system is a problem that was brought up by participants, both the older homeless and providers, frequently. Besides the desire voiced by providers for more staff who are specialized in benefits, provider interviews led to mention of new models that are seeking to overcome this problem throughout the country. Some these programs were contacted after interviews were completed and the researchers learned of some of the innovative methods they are using to achieve success when working with individuals over 50. For one program, success was attributed to the ability to focus on the increased difficulty in finding employment or obtaining re-training – a problem generally recognized as legitimate by Social Security. Legal assistance programs were also reported as successful in helping people to obtain benefits after other failed attempts. These programs focus their success on their ability to reconstruct detailed client histories, having access to funding for obtaining appropriate documentation, the participation of medical experts who are willing to conduct more in-depth assessments than homeless individuals would typically receive, and the authority given to key social security staff to provide assistance for individuals based on "presumed disability" while awaiting a formal diagnosis.

Limitations

The major limitations of this study are related to the sampling process and weaknesses in the administrative data collected from homeless service organizations. While a convenience sample was used, the list of agencies that participants eventually came from represented the "major players" of homeless services in the city of Chicago, and data collected can be reasoned to be representative of the entire system. The Researchers also made every attempt to gain participation from agencies and individuals who represented unique situations, that is, services and/or populations, if they were known. The weakness of the data collected from agencies represented the lack of understanding of the usefulness of data within social service organizations. In most instances databases only existed because they were needed for providing required information to funders; these databases usually only reflected the exact information needed for these funding purposes. Regardless of the weaknesses of the data, the study has strengths that cannot be overlooked. The survey data analyzed from the Roundtable study was from a representative sample. Also, triangulation of data showed agreement between the various sources that helped to define the sweeping issues of the older homeless, and this cannot be overlooked.

Due to a lack of comparable data, the health problems of the older homeless and those 50–64 in the general population could not be investigated for this chapter. Future research needs to take this issue into consideration in order to find applicable methods of assessing the similarities and differences between these two groups.

CONCLUSIONS

Those ages 50–64 are often not considered when designing or providing health care services for homeless individuals. Traditionally, homeless services have been designed with the needs of the younger homeless in mind, while public benefits are often difficult for those under 64 to qualify for. Issues such as these pose problems for the older homeless that have effects on the entire society because of the significant cost they impose on the health care system, and these issues need to be better understood.

After outlining previous research, this chapter connected findings from a study on the older homeless in Chicago to those found in the previous literature. These findings described the quantity and type of health care problems in this population as well as the barriers they face in obtaining health care services. After outlining these findings, the chapter proposed some possible ways that the health care needs of the older homeless can be better addressed through policy and program initiatives that seek to understand the unique issues that result from the intersection of age and homelessness.

While already significant, the impact the older homeless will have on the resources of homeless service and health care systems in the future will be overwhelming considering the trends in growth that this and previous studies have shown. These trends highlight the need to better understand the issues that this population faces so that they can be better met.

NOTE

1. The reason for defining the older homeless as those 50–64 and not 50 and older is due to the issues that this group faces which are uniquely different from those both younger and older.

REFERENCES

Brickner, P. W., & Scanlan, B. C. (1990). Health care for homeless persons: Creation and implementation of a program. In: P. W. Brickner, L. K. Schafer, B. A. Conanan, M. Savarese & B. C. Scanlan (Eds), *Under the safety net: The health and social welfare of the homeless in the United States* (pp. 3–14). New York, NY: WW Norton and Company.

Burt, M., Laudan, A., & Lee, E. (2001). *Helping America's homeless: Emergency shelter or affordable housing?* Washington, DC: The Urban Institute Press.

Cohen, C. I. (1999). Aging and homelessness. *The Gerontologist, 39*, 5–14.

Cohen, C. I., & Skolovsky, J. (1989). *Old men of the bowery*. New York: Guilford Press.

Cohen, C. I., Teresi, J., & Holmes, D. (1988). Survival strategies of older homeless men. *The Gerontologist, 28*, 58–65.

Crane, M., & Warnes, A. (2001). Older people and homelessness prevalence and causes. *Top Geriatric Rehabilitation, 16*, 1–4.

Crane, M., & Warnes, A. M. (2005). Responding to the needs of older homeless people. *Innovation, 18*, 137–152.

Dennis, D. L., Levine, I. S., & Osher, F. C. (1991). The physical and mental health status of homeless adults. *Housing Policy Debate, 2*, 815–835.

Dickey, B., Normand, S.-L. T., Weiss, R. D., Drake, R. E., & Azenie, H. (2002). Medical morbidity, mental illness, and substance use disorders. *Psychiatric Services, 53*, 861–867.

Dietz, T. L., & Wright, J. D. (2003). Homelessness among the elderly. In: *The encyclopedia of retirement and finance* (pp. 381–386). Westport, CT: Greenwood Press.

Gallagher, T., Andersen, R. M., Kogel, P., & Gelberg, L. (1997). Determinants of regular source of care among homeless adults in Los Angeles. *Medical Care, 35*, 814–830.

Gelberg, L., Andersen, R. M., & Leake, B. D. (2002). The behavioral model for vulnerable populations: Application to medical care use and outcomes for homeless people. *Health Services Research, 34*, 1273–1302.

Gelberg, L., Linn, L. S., & Mayer-Oakes, S. A. (1990). Differences in health status between older and younger homeless adults. *Journal of the American Geriatrics Society, 38*, 1220–1229.

Hahn, J. A., Kushel, M. B., Bangsberg, D. R., Riley, E., & Moss, A. R. (2005). Brief report: The aging of the homeless population – fourteen-year trends in San Francisco. *Journal of Internal Medicine, 21*, 775–778.

Han, B., Wells, B. L., & Taylor, A. M. (2003). Use of the health care for the homeless program services and other health care services by homeless adults. *Journal of Health Care for the Poor and Underserved, 14*, 87–99.

Hatchett, B. F. (2004). Homelessness among older adults in a Texas border town. *Journal of Aging and Social Policy, 16*, 35–57.

Hecht, L., & Coyle, B. (2001). Elderly homeless: A comparison of older and younger adult emergency shelter seekers in Bakersfield, California. *American Behavioral Scientist, 45*, 66–79.

Illinois Regional Roundtable on Homelessness. (2002). *Regional roundtable on homelessness: Homeless needs assessment project.* Illinois Regional Continuum of Care Roundtable.

Institute of Medicine. (2003). *Hidden costs, values lost: Uninsurance in America.* Washington, DC: National Academy Press.

Kaiser Family Foundation. (2007). The uninsured, a primer: Key facts about Americans without health insurance. Retrieved March 7, 2008 (http://www.kff.org/uninsured/upload/7451-03.pdf).

Kushel, M. B., Vittinghoff, E., & Hass, J. S. (2001). Factors associated with the health care utilization of homeless persons. *Journal of the American Medical Association, 285*, 200–206.

Kutza, E. A., & Keigher, S. M. (1991). The elderly "new homeless": An emerging population at risk. *Social Work, 36*, 288–293.

North, C. S., Eyrich, K. M., Pollio, D. E., & Spitznagel, E. L. (2004). Are rates of psychiatric disorders in the homeless population changing? *American Journal of Public Health, 94*, 103–108.

Padgett, D., Struening, E. L., & Andrews, H. (1990). Factors affecting the use of medical, mental health, alcohol and drug treatment services by homeless adults. *Medical Care, 28*, 805–820.

Resenbaum, S., & Zuvekas, A. (1995). Healthcare use by homeless persons: Implications for public policy. *Health Services Research, 34*, 1303–1305.

Rossi, P. H. (1989). *Down and out in America: The origins of homelessness.* Chicago, IL: University of Chicago Press.

Sachs-Ericsson, N., Wise, E., Debrody, C. P., & Paniucki, H. B. (1999). Health problems and service utilization in the homeless. *Journal of Health Care for the Poor and Underserved, 10*, 443–452.

Scharer, L. K., Berson, A., & Brickner, P. W. (1990). Lack of housing and its impact on human health: A service perspective. *Bulletin of the New York Academy of Medicine, 66*, 515–525.

Smith, J. L. (2003). *Aging and homelessness: Research on people age 50 and older who are homeless or at-risk of homelessness in the Chicago region.* UIC Urban Planning and Policy Program, 2002. Retrieved February 12, 2008 (http://www.heartlandalliance.org/maip/documents/AgingandHomelessness_000.pdf).

The Commonwealth Fund. (2003). The costs and consequences of being uninsured. In the Literature. Retrieved March 7, 2008 (http://www.commonwealthfund.org/usr_doc/davis_consequences_itl_663.pdf?section = 4039).

THE URBANIZATION OF POVERTY AND URBAN SLUM PREVALENCE: THE IMPACT OF THE BUILT ENVIRONMENT ON POPULATION-LEVEL PATTERNS OF SOCIAL WELL-BEING IN THE LESS DEVELOPED COUNTRIES

James Rice

ABSTRACT

The urbanization of poverty is a structural trend embodied in the sprawling urban slums of the developing countries. It remains a largely unacknowledged dynamic. This is particularly true in terms of the population-level patterns of social well-being derived from urban slum prevalence or proportion of the total population living in urban slum conditions. In particular, there is increasing evidence of an "urban penalty" wherein urban slum dwellers exhibit poorer health outcomes than non-slum urban residents and even rural populations. We articulate the proposition that urban slum prevalence is a key factor shaping

Care for Major Health Problems and Population Health Concerns:
Impacts on Patients, Providers and Policy
Research in the Sociology of Health Care, Volume 26, 205–234
Copyright © 2008 by Emerald Group Publishing Limited
All rights of reproduction in any form reserved
ISSN: 0275-4959/doi:10.1016/S0275-4959(08)26010-2

population-level rates of social well-being in the developing countries, measured at the national level. Further, we develop the proposition drawn from political economy of health theorization suggesting cross-national dependency relations substantially influence urban slum conditions. In turn, the structural dynamics of the world economy underlie urban slum prevalence which itself has a direct influence on population-level patterns of social well-being as measured by infant and under-five mortality, maternal mortality, and life expectancy at birth. We conclude by arguing for greater empirical attention focusing upon the consequences of dependency relations as expressed in the built urban environment and the impact of urban slum prevalence as a key social condition impacting well-being in the less developed countries.

INTRODUCTION

Urban residents are frequently conceptualized as healthier, better educated, and more prosperous than their rural counterparts and urbanization in general is often assumed to be a positive step towards social and economic development. There is evidence, however, of an increasing "urban penalty" reflected in socio-spatial health disparities between urban slum residents and both non-slum urban residents and even rural populations within the developing countries [United Nations Human Settlements Programme (UN-HABITAT), 2006].

The ascendance of urban slums characterized by overcrowding and inadequate access to basic public services is one of the most notable trends of the past several decades and promises to remain so far into the 21st century. As Bolay (2006) notes, the proliferation of urban slum conditions is not an anomaly or transient phenomenon but the very essence of contemporary urbanization processes in the less developed countries. It is not simply the consequence of population growth. It is also tied to the increasing urbanization of poverty or spatial relocation of deprivation driven by the "push" of rural out-migration without the consequent urban "pull" of parallel industrialization and economic growth (UN-HABITAT, 2003a). In turn, the contradictory processes of economic globalization are increasingly manifest within the urban areas of the developing countries. Enclaves of modern office buildings and gated, up-scale communities surrounded by sprawling slums are the visible expression of such contradictions.

There is a segment of humanity nearly one billion strong "warehoused" in the teeming urban slums of the developing countries and lacking suitable avenues of escape (Davis, 2006). This "concentration of disadvantage" (Vlahov et al., 2007, p. i16), moreover, constitutes an increasingly prominent structural characteristic shaping population-level patterns of health and illness. To understand morbidity and mortality rates and patterns in the developing countries increasingly requires consideration of the expanding prevalence of urban slums.

Poverty, overcrowding, malnutrition, insufficient garbage disposal, lack of adequate water drainage, and unsafe drinking water and sanitation coalesce around the social organization of marginalized populations in urban slums. Overall slum dwellers are more likely to die earlier, experience greater malnutrition and hunger, exhibit higher diseases rates, attain less education, and have fewer employment opportunities than urban residents living outside the slums (UN-HABITAT, 2006). Even more striking is the accumulating evidence urban slum residents often exhibit poorer health and lower literacy and economic opportunities than rural residents (UN-HABITAT, 2006). Women living in slums are more likely to contract HIV/AIDS than their rural counterparts and in many sub-Saharan African countries slum residents' exhibit rates of HIV prevalence substantially higher than rural populations (UN-HABITAT, 2006). Child malnutrition within many urban slums is comparable to that observed in rural areas and the incidence of waterborne diseases and respiratory illnesses is often higher (UN-HABITAT, 2006).

The intent of the present chapter is to articulate the proposition that urban slum prevalence is a key factor or social-organizational pattern shaping population-level rates of social well-being in the less developed countries (LDCs) measured at the national level.[1] Such an urban penalty is clearly recognizable in relation to non-slum urban residents; we suggest, however, the urban penalty derived from the expansion of urban slum conditions has become so prominent that it is also recognizable measured at the national level, a consideration generally overlooked in the research literature. Further, we outline the proposition that dependency relations as embodied through external debt burden promote the formulation of urban slum conditions. The analyses presented are intended to be suggestive of the validity of these propositions and agitate for greater empirical attention to the contradictions of urban social organization embodied in the ascendance of urban slum conditions and expressed through variance in population-level measures of social well-being.

We begin by reviewing the criteria for delineating slum versus non-slum urban households and highlight regional trends in slum relative to urban growth. Second, we examine the contradictions of urban social organization that increasingly call into question the assumption that urbanization is an unproblematic step on the path towards social and economic development. Third, we argue deep-seated social factors in general and political economy of health theorization in particular are valuable frameworks for developing a more comprehensive understanding of the social production of variant patterns of health and illness as a consequence of the urbanization of poverty. Fourth, we identify a number of implications derived from the recognition of urban slum prevalence as a factor shaping patterns of health and illness and conclude by highlighting future research concerns.

THE ASCENDANCE OF URBAN SLUMS IN THE DEVELOPING WORLD: AN OVERVIEW

A slum constitutes, in general terms, a densely populated area exhibiting substandard housing and standard of living (UN-HABITAT, 2003b). In concrete terms, Table 1 outlines the criteria established by UN-HABITAT to delineate slum versus non-slum urban households. The designation is based on the absence of one or more of the following: improved water supply, improved sanitation, sufficient living area, durability of construction, and security of tenure.[2] The degree of deprivation is predicated upon how many of the criteria highlighted in Table 1 are absent. Lack of access to improved water and sanitation are the most common indicators of urban slum residence in the developing countries (UN-HABITAT, 2003a). Lack of durability of construction and overcrowding are the next most common indicators. Approximately one-fifth of urban slums worldwide are extremely deprived as indicated by the absence of three or more of the established standards (UN-HABITAT, 2007a).

The designation "improved" refers to water and sanitation provisioning that meet particular criteria. The standards measure both quantity and source protection of drinking water and the degree to which sanitation facilities reduce the chances of individuals coming into contact with human excreta and thereby a common pathway of disease transmission. Improved sources are argued to provide sufficient quantities of water to maintain hygiene and insure safer drinking water and more sanitary methods of excreta disposal than unimproved services.[3]

Table 1. Criteria for Delineating Slum and Non-Slum Urban Households.

An urban household is defined as a slum dwelling if it lacks one or more of the following:

1. *Access to an Improved Water Supply*: That provides a sufficient quantity of water for family use (at least 20 liters/person/day), at an affordable price (less than 10 percent of total household income), without requiring extreme effort to obtain (less than 1 hour a day for the minimum sufficient quantity). In addition, an improved water supply consists of the following delivery systems:

- Piped connection to house or plot
- Public stand pipe serving no more than five households
- Bore hole
- Protected dug well
- Protected spring
- Rain water collection.

2. *Access to Improved Sanitation*: Consisting of a private or public toilet shared between a reasonable number of people. Improved sanitation consists of the following services:

- Direct connection to public sewer
- Direct connection to a septic tank
- Pour flush latrine
- Ventilated pit latrine.

3. *Sufficient Living Area*: Overcrowding is defined as three or more people per habitable room (minimum of 4 square meters of space).

4. *Durability of Construction*: A dwelling is defined as durable if it is built in a non-hazardous location and exhibits structural qualities adequate to protect its inhabitants from the extremes of climatic conditions, including rain, heat, cold, and humidity. A non-hazardous location is defined as:

- The dwelling is not located on or near toxic waste
- The dwelling is not located in a flood plain
- The dwelling is not located on a steep slope
- The dwelling is not located in a dangerous right of way (rail, highway, airport, power lines).

Assessment of structural quality is shaped by prevailing local conditions and therefore exhibits considerable variability in definition. An earthen floor, for example, may be defined as durable in some countries but un-durable in other countries relative to broader prevailing living conditions. An underlying criterion, in turn, for assessing durability of construction is the degree to which a dwelling exhibits a permanency of structure in terms of the walls, roof, and floor in manner that protects inhabitants from the weather without need for major repair.

5. *Security of Tenure*: Residents have protection against arbitrary and/or unlawful eviction.

Source: Adapted from UN-HABITAT (2003a).

Durability of construction refers to both the materials utilized and the location in which the household is situated relative to common hazards found in the urban environment. Deficient housing complicates water, sanitation, and food preparation and storage needs (Brown, 2003). Further, urban slum dwellers often occupy the most marginalized and least economically productive land and therefore live coincident to a number of geologic and industrial hazards, increasing exposure to floods, landslides, and pollution (Davis, 2006; Satterthwaite, 1993).

Sufficient living area is of concern as overcrowding makes adequate hygienic practices to maintain health increasingly problematic at the household and community level. Overcrowding makes urban residents vulnerable to a litany of communicable diseases that include tuberculosis, acute respiratory infections, and meningitis (Sclar, Garau, & Carolini, 2005). The higher prevalence of malnutrition within urban slums, moreover, facilitates the transmission of disease due to lowered immunity among overcrowded slum populations (Sclar et al., 2005).

Security of tenure refers to the degree to which residents are protected against arbitrary and/or unlawful eviction (UN-HABITAT, 2003a). Many slum households do not hold formal legal title to the land upon which they reside or legally enforceable agreements constituting proof of tenure arrangements (UN-HABITAT, 2003a, 2003b). Frequently slums consist of illegally or informally occupied areas of land (Bolay, 2006; Davis, 2006; UN-HABITAT, 2003a, 2003b). Many are characterized by an uncertain and precarious existence as eviction is an ever-present threat and there exist, in turn, substantial disincentives to individual and community investment in upgrading living conditions (Bolay, 2006).

It is estimated that 920 million people, about one-third of the world's total urban population, live in slums in 2001, the vast majority located in the LDCs (UN-HABITAT, 2003a).[4] Further, the proportion of total and urban populations living in slums is projected to increase steadily in the coming decades, an estimated 27 million new slum dwellers annually over the period 2000–2020 (UN-HABITAT, 2006). Worldwide the aggregate urban slum population grew 36 percent in the 1990s (UN-HABITAT, 2003b). At the current pace it is estimated that over the next 30 years the overall number worldwide will increase to over 2 billion (UN-HABITAT, 2003b).

Fig. 1 illustrates the annual growth of *aggregate* urban slum populations relative to aggregate urban population growth from 1990 to 2001 by region.[5] Sub-Saharan Africa exhibits the fastest urbanization and slum growth over the period. Moreover, virtually all of the urban growth consists of slum formation or expansion. From 1990 to 2001 the slum population in sub-Saharan Africa

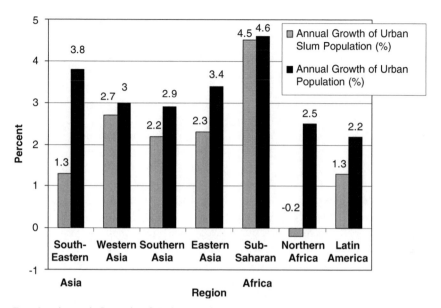

Fig. 1. Annual Growth of Urban and Slum Populations 1990–2001 by Region. *Data source:* UN-HABITAT (2007b). Figure is based on the 165 countries listed in Table A1 in the Appendix.

grew by 64 percent (UN-HABITAT, 2007b); this equates to an annual average growth rate of 4.58 percent, higher than the total population growth rate over the period. At this pace it is estimated the slums in sub-Saharan Africa will double from 2001 to 2016 (UN-HABITAT, 2007b).

Western Asia also exhibits roughly parallel slum and urban growth from 1990 to 2001 such that most urban growth is occurring in the slums or is expressed as slum formation. Overall, the urban slum population expanded by 40 percent over the period in Western Asia. Other areas of the continent are characterized by lower slum growth relative to urban growth. However, in terms of absolute numbers Southern and Eastern Asia is characterized by the greatest number of urban slum residents as a proportion of the world total in 2001. India, for example, has 158 million slum dwellers and China has 178 million, together accounting for one-third of the world total (UN-HABITAT, 2003a). Slum growth relative to urban growth overall was also lower within Latin American and the Caribbean. Aggregate slum population growth in the region averaged 15 percent over the period (UN-HABITAT, 2003a).

The only developing region to experience a decline in the population living in slums from 1990 to 2001 and a consequent increase in urban quality of life was Northern Africa. A recent United Nations report credits governmental efforts to upgrade slums and prevent their formation as one of the main factors underlying this decline (UN-HABITAT, 2006).

Fig. 2 highlights urban slum intensity or the proportion of *urban* populations living in slum conditions in 2001 by region. Sub-Saharan African countries are characterized by the greatest overall mean urban slum intensity at 71.9 percent. This illustrates that although the mass or magnitude of urban slum residents as a proportion of the world total is highest in Asia the concentration of slum residents as a proportion of the urban population is highest in sub-Saharan Africa. Within many sub-Saharan countries, in turn, a clear majority of the urban population lives in slum conditions. In some countries virtually the entire urban population lives in slum conditions. For example, urban slum intensity in Ethiopia is 99.4 percent, in Chad it is 99.1 percent, and in Somalia and Sierra Leone 97.1 and 95.8 percent of the urban population reside in slum conditions (UN-HABITAT, 2003a). The slums in sub-Saharan Africa, moreover, are the most disadvantaged in the world relative to the criteria outlined in Table 1 (UN-HABITAT, 2007a).

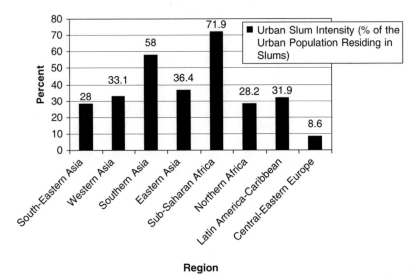

Fig. 2. Urban Slum Prevalence 2001 by Region. *Data source:* UN-HABITAT (2003a). Figure is based on the 165 countries listed in Table A1 in the Appendix.

Southern Asia is also characterized by a clear majority of urban residents living in slum conditions at 58 percent. Within other regions of the world roughly one-third of the urban population lives in slum conditions. The notable exception is Central-Eastern European countries which illustrate a much lower proportion on average.

The growth of slums is a reflection of the accelerating urbanization of poverty or shifting of deprivation within LDCs to urban contexts (UN-HABITAT, 2003b). This reorganization is highlighted by the increasingly problematic intersection between the built and biophysical environments expressed in urban slum conditions. It is not simply the lack of services that presents unique health challenges but lack of services concurrent with densely populated areas frequently located directly upon or proximate to toxic and hazardous areas of land. Although they often border and even roughly encircle urban areas, typically slums are socially, politically, and economically isolated from the broader urban setting and their residents lack access to many formal institutions in society (UN-HABITAT, 2003b). There are generally considerable barriers, in turn, to accessing quality health care and emergency services for slum dwellers (Sclar et al., 2005).

URBAN SOCIAL ORGANIZATION IN THE DEVELOPING COUNTRIES: EXAMINING THE CONUNDRUM

As Vlahov et al. (2007) observe, the higher the proportion of a country urbanized or urbanicity the higher that country typically ranks in terms of social well-being measured at the national level. However, the higher the levels of urbanization, or processes of urban reorganization and change, the lower are social well-being achievements on average.[6] This conundrum is a reflection of fact that despite the numerous advantages offered by urban social organization the rapidity of urbanization creates enormous challenges. Such challenges, moreover, appear to increasingly outweigh the advantages for marginalized segments of the urban population.

Urban slum prevalence is the spatial and material outcome of urbanization processes enacted within a context of lack of employment, housing, and basic public services. And it is the unprecedented growth of urban slums that threatens to undercut the anticipated social well-being advantages of urban life in ways that many researchers have not yet fully considered.

Table 2 includes the Pearson bivariate and partial correlation coefficients between national-level measures of social well-being and extent of urban social organization defined as the percent of the population living in urban areas and urban slum prevalence or proportion of the total population living in urban slums conditions.[7] The top-third of Table 2 illustrates the juxtaposition between urbanicity and level of urban slum prevalence.

Table 2. Urban Characteristics and Social Well-Being Correlation Coefficients.

	Urban Population 2000 (%)	Urban Slum Prevalence 2001 (%)
Bivariate Correlation Coefficients		
Infant Mortality Rate 2005	−.602***	.452***
Under-five Mortality Rate 2005	−.612***	.447***
Maternal Mortality Rate 2005	−.605***	.458***
Life Expectancy at Birth 2005	.560***	−.289**
Gender Development Index 2005	.681***	−.324***
Partial Correlation Coefficients Controlling for GDP Per Capita 2000		
Infant Mortality Rate 2005	−.058	.544***
Under-five Mortality Rate 2005	−.055	.549***
Maternal Mortality Rate 2005	−.164	.515***
Life Expectancy at Birth 2005	.183	−.270**
Gender Development Index 2005	.138	−.387***
Partial Correlation Coefficients Controlling for GDP Per Capita 2000 and Urban Population Growth 1990–2003 (Average Annual %)		
Infant Mortality Rate 2005	.077	.431***
Under-five Mortality Rate 2005	.089	.433***
Maternal Mortality Rate 2005	.004	.366***
Life Expectancy at Birth 2005	.104	−.131
Gender Development Index 2005	.009	−.212*

$^*p < .05$; $^{**}p < .01$; $^{***}p < .001$ (two-tailed tests).
Note: Pearson correlation coefficients are based on all less developed countries with available data on all variables included in Table 2. This consists of the 98 countries listed in Table A1 in the Appendix. Infant mortality, child mortality, and life expectancy data source: UNICEF (2007). Maternal mortality data source: World Health Organization (WHO) (2007). GDP per capita data source: World Bank (2006b). Urbanization data source: World Bank (2005). Urban slum prevalence refers to the percent of the total population living in urban slum conditions in 2001. Data is obtained from UN-HABITAT (2003a). To avoid the influence of outlying data points we examined the standardized residuals of all cases reported in Table 2. No data points exhibited a standardized residual greater or lesser than 3 standard deviations. Consistent with assumptions underlying the statistical significance tests reported, we performed natural log transformations on those measures with evidence of non-normal distributions. The following are in natural log form: infant mortality, under-five mortality, maternal mortality, life expectancy at birth, gender development index, and GDP per capita.

Infant, child, and maternal mortality exhibit a strong and statistically significant *negative* association with level of urbanicity. This suggests developing countries characterized by a greater proportion of their population living in urban areas exhibit lower rates of mortality. Further, proportion of the population residing in urban areas is associated with longer life expectancy at birth.

The gender development index (GDI) is a composite indicator comprised of four components measuring the well-being of women relative to that of men. These include: life expectancy, literacy rates, education enrollment rates, and income ratio. Higher scores on the GDI indicate greater parity between women and men. Of note, urban population level has a beneficial positive correlation with the gender development index. This implies more urbanized developing countries are characterized by greater parity between men and women.

In contrast, urban slum prevalence exhibits a strong *positive* correlation with infant, child, and maternal mortality. Developing countries characterized by greater proportions of their population living in urban slum conditions exhibit higher mortality levels. Further, urban slum prevalence is strongly correlated with declining life expectancy at birth. This provides population-level evidence that indeed the prevalence of urban slum conditions has an influence on mortality.

In turn, urban slum prevalence is associated with declining gender parity. This in and of itself is relevant to consideration of infant, child, and maternal mortality as the empowerment of women has a direct influence on their own morbidity and mortality and that of children (Scanlan, 2004; Shen & Williamson, 1997, 1999, 2001). The empowerment of women contributes to basic measures of social well-being as it enhances their knowledge, skills, and income that promote access to and management of health information and services (Caldwell, 1990; Shen & Williamson, 1999; Wickrama & Lorenz, 2002). Caldwell (1990) argues female education, for example, enhances not simply women's status relative to men and therefore access to health services but management and application of the information and services received. He notes educated women tend to engage in greater preventative measures to keep children from becoming sick and more effective and assertive efforts to treat a child after they have fallen ill.

The deleterious association between urban slum prevalence and gender parity is consistent with the contention that the increasing urbanization of poverty is simultaneously the expanding feminization of poverty (UN-HABITAT, 2003b). Women bear a disproportionate burden as a consequence of rapid urbanization as they are the most vulnerable of urban slum residents in terms of personal safety, access to economic opportunities, and access to basic public services (UN-HABITAT, 2003b). Women headed households are increasingly common within urban slums and legal and/or cultural traditions often restrict their housing options both within and outside urban slum areas as they frequently do not have the opportunity to attain legal land titles (UN-HABITAT, 2003a, 2003b). Women-headed households, for example, account for 30 percent or more of the households within low-income, primarily slum, urban areas in Africa (UN-HABITAT, 2003b).

More compelling is the association between proportion of the population living in urban areas and urban slum prevalence with social well-being net the influence of economic development, which arguably is strongly linked to all of the above. The middle-third of Table 2 includes the partial correlation coefficients controlling for GDP per capita. The results illustrate urbanicity is no longer correlated with any of the social well-being measures or gender development at a statistically significant level net the influence of economic development. Conversely, urban slum prevalence is characterized by strong positive associations with infant, child, and maternal mortality even after controlling for GDP per capita. Further, developing countries with greater urban slum conditions exhibit lower life expectancy at birth and lower gender parity net level of economic development.

The partial correlation coefficient results highlighted in the middle-third of Table 2 suggest the deleterious association of urban slum prevalence and social well-being cannot simply be equated with poverty. In turn, these results lend credence to Krieger's (2001a, p. 899) assertion: "Context and level matter: poor people living in poor neighborhoods are likely to have poorer health than equally poor people living in more affluent neighbor-hoods." This is an assertion Engels (1968[1845]) proffered more than 150 years ago in his examination of the living conditions of the English working class but bears repeating in relation to the burgeoning urban slums of the developing countries. Context matters – particularly for marginalized segments of a population.

The bottom-third of Table 2 includes partial correlation coefficients net the influence of GDP per capita and urbanization or urban change over the period 1990–2003. The results demonstrate urban slum prevalence exhibits deleterious associations with the social well-being measures at a statistically significant level net economic development and urbanization, with the exception of the life expectancy at birth measure. This is notable as it suggests the contradictory dynamics characterizing urban social organiza-tion are not simply the consequence of the rapidity of urban change. The rapidity of urban change fuels the ascendance of urban slums. It is the prevalence of urban slums, however, that has a substantial direct association with national-level measures of social well-being not the movement of people in and out of urban areas per se.

The non-significance of the correlation between urban slum prevalence and life expectancy at birth within the bottom-third of Table 2 is consistent with the differing etiological and temporal dynamics that plausibly link urban slum conditions and the constituent social well-being measures. A central challenge facing researchers attempting to model the effects of social determinants and health and illness concerns the temporal dynamics connecting acute or chronic exposure to unhealthy conditions and the latency period associated with consequent morbidity and mortality (Krieger, 1999). The temporal plausibility or inference of concurrent effect between urban slum prevalence and life expectancy at birth is problematic relative to the other social well-being measures in Table 2 given individuals move in and out of different residential settings over their lifetime and mortality may be the consequence of disease of short or long latency periods. Infant, child, and maternal mortality are events exhibiting more truncated, circumscribed temporal dynamics and the inference of an association with urban slum conditions, therefore, is more plausible. Indeed, the partial correlation coefficients highlighted in the bottom-third of Table 2 mirror such anticipated temporal and etiological dynamics.

The deleterious consequences of urban slum prevalence may be particularly apparent through examination of the effects upon children. The five illnesses at the root of a majority of child deaths in the developing countries include pneumonia, diarrhea, malaria, measles, and HIV/AIDS (UN-HABITAT, 2007c). Each is prevalent in many urban slums due primarily to substandard living conditions and overcrowding (UN-HABITAT, 2007c). Inadequate access to clean water and sanitation, in particular, are a direct cause of a substantial proportion of deaths of children under-five annually [United Nations Development Programme (UNDP), 2006]. Poor water quality and quantity and inadequate sanitation are linked to a number of waterborne and water-washed diseases (UNDP, 2006). Further, many slum children are malnourished, increasing their susceptibility to illness (Bartlett, 2003; Ghosh & Shah, 2004; Wagstaff, Bustreo, Bryce, & Claeson, 2004). Children living in urban slums in India, for example, are on average more malnourished than non-slum urban and even rural children (Ghosh & Shah, 2004). Further, research suggests neonatal mortality in urban slums is linked to home deliveries, low birth weight, delay in seeking medical attention, and the lack of or inappropriate medical treatment and services (Fernandez, Mondkar, & Mathai, 2003).

Greater morbidity and mortality among urban slum children are not simply the consequence of household level deficiencies but also include health issues arising within the context of the broader slum settlement (Agarwal & Taneja, 2005; Awasthi & Agarwal, 2003; Bartlett, 2003). Inadequate water drainage and waste removal often creates areas of contamination extending throughout the surrounding community (Bartlett, 2003). In turn, many slums lack safe places for children to play outdoors (Bartlett, 2003; Satterthwaite, 1993). Moreover, there is litany of indoor and outdoor chemical pollutants frequently encountered in low-income urban areas that compromise the health of children (Satterthwaite, 1993).

Table 3 highlights the 15 overachieving and underachieving LDCs in terms of under-five mortality in 2005 relative to level of GDP per capita in 2000. The rankings are derived by regressing child mortality on GDP per capita and then examining the unstandardized residuals. The residuals indicate the observed level of under-five mortality relative to that predicted by regression upon GDP per capita. Low unstandardized residuals signify countries with lower child mortality than expected given their level of GDP per capita. High residuals indicate countries with greater child mortality than expected given their per capita income level.

The top 15 overachieving countries exhibit a mean urban slum prevalence of 5.9 percent. The top 15 underachieving countries are characterized by a much higher proportion of their total population living in urban slum conditions at an average of 28.4 percent, nearly 5 times higher than the best performing LDCs. The underachieving countries are characterized by levels of child mortality unexpected given their level of economic development; and, they exhibit substantially greater urban slum conditions. In turn, Table 3 suggests urban slum prevalence has a direct influence on child mortality levels among the best and worst performing LDCs above and beyond the influence of income per capita.

Gabon and Congo are characterized by a majority of their total population living in urban slum conditions; within several other underachieving countries the proportion of the population living in urban slum conditions is approximately one-third. Of note, 12 of the 15 worst performing LDCs are sub-Saharan African countries. Indeed, sub-Saharan Africa has the highest child mortality rates of any region in the world (Mogford, 2004; UNICEF, 2007). Since the 1990s reduction in under-five mortality within many sub-Saharan African countries has stagnated and even reversed course (Mogford, 2004). Further, over the period 1990–2001 the aggregate urban slum population in sub-Saharan Africa expanded by 64 percent, the fastest growth rate of any region in the world (UN-HABITAT, 2007b).

Table 3. Relative Child Mortality Rate 2005: Overachieving and Underachieving Countries.

Country	Residual	Urban Slum Prevalence (%)	Country	Residual	Urban Slum Prevalence (%)
Top 15 Overachievers			*Top 15 Underachievers*		
1. Moldova	−1.87	12.8	1. Botswana	1.86	30
2. Vietnam	−1.49	11.6	2. Gabon	1.65	54.5
3. Sri Lanka	−1.32	3.1	3. Angola	1.47	29
4. Czech Republic	−1.27	4.2	4. South Africa	1.15	19.6
5. Ukraine	−1.26	4.1	5. Côte d'Ivoire	1.11	29.9
6. Belarus	−1.19	3.9	6. Cameroon	.91	33.3
7. Syria	−1.04	5.4	7. Nigeria	.83	35.6
8. Croatia	−.91	4.5	8. Congo	.79	59.5
9. Estonia	−.91	8.5	9. Zimbabwe	.72	1.2
10. Slovakia	−.85	3.2	10. Namibia	.72	11.9
11. Armenia	−.79	1.3	11. Mexico	.71	14.6
12. Albania	−.79	3	12. Lebanon	.68	45.1
13. Tajikistan	−.79	15.5	13. Kazakhstan	.61	16.6
14. Bulgaria	−.77	3.8	14. Lesotho	.58	16.4
15. Hungary	−.71	3.6	15. Zambia	.56	29.4
Mean		*5.9*	*Mean*		*28.4*
Median		*4.1*	*Median*		*29.4*

Note: Illustrated above are the top 15 overachieving and underachieving countries based on examination of child mortality rate relative to level of GDP per capita. Table includes unstandardized residuals derived from the regression of under-five mortality rate 2005 (natural log) on GDP per capita 2000 (natural log). Countries with the lowest residuals have low child mortality relative to their GDP per capita; those with the highest residuals have high child mortality relative to their GDP per capita. Urban slum prevalence refers to the percent of the total population living in urban slum conditions in 2001. Data is obtained from UN-HABITAT (2003a). Income data obtained from World Bank (2006b). Table is based on analysis of the 98 countries listed in Table A1 in the Appendix.

DEPENDENCY RELATIONS AND THE PROLIFERATION OF URBAN SLUMS IN THE DEVELOPING COUNTRIES

Epidemiological studies have greatly contributed to the identification of the individual-level risk factors shaping the incidence of morbidity and mortality, but a renewed emphasis on the identification of "basic social conditions" is crucial to delineating the "distal" or contextual determinants that further constitute fundamental causes of health or illness (Link & Phelan, 1995, p. 80, 1996); at issue are the factors shaping *susceptibility to* rather than the biomedical *mechanisms of* disease causation per se (Krieger, 2001b). The challenge, in turn, is to recognize the manner in which "societies shape patterns of disease" (Link & Phelan, 1996, p. 471; Waitzkin, 1981).

As McKinlay (1981) notes, a majority of resources and attention devoted to public health concerns are applied downstream or in reference to problem-solving interventions designed to address various, and shifting, health issues. Often the real and more enduring problems, however, exist upstream in terms of the structure or access and adequacy of health care provisioning and the social context in which different segments of a population live their lives, thus shaping differential exposure to risk (McKinlay, 1981).

Drawing from the identification of upstream, basic social conditions, we suggest the recognition of urban slum prevalence is a key dimension shaping social well-being in the less developed countries and one avenue whereby social-organizational patterns shape the incidence of morbidity and mortality. Further, we draw from the political economy of health theoretical perspective in particular to suggest health and illness is shaped not simply by endogenous societal dynamics but also the exogenous interrelationships between societies. Indeed, the social context wherein an individual's relationships to others and to domestic institutional health care services is enacted is important in understanding differential morbidity and mortality; the form and dynamics of the world economy, moreover, shape such lower-scale social considerations.

Political economy of health theorization focuses on the macro-comparative effects upon health and illness of hierarchical political-economic relations within the world economy (Morgan, 1987; Waitzkin, 1981). Dependency and world-systems researchers argue development and underdevelopment are mutually constituted through the continual reproduction of the structural parameters and momentum of the world economy, a consequence of cross-national political-economic interdependencies (Chase-Dunn, 1989; Frank, 1966; Wallerstein, 1974). As Amin (1974) observes, underdevelopment is not synonymous with poverty. It is characterized by economic, social, and political structural patterns within dependent countries congruent with narrow exogenous interests but generally incongruent with broader development goals. Underdevelopment, moreover, is reflected in population-level patterns of health and illness (Elling, 1981; Turshen, 1977).

Drawing from the political economy of health perspective, urban slum prevalence is arguably driven by dependency relations enacted at a cross-national scale – particularly debt dependency. Indeed, urban slum prevalence is potentially one expression of the overdevelopment-under-development dynamics enacted through the structural momentum of the world economy. The material conditions in which marginalized segments of a population live is impacted by the material relations of production that give form to the modern world-system. Central to such processes is the external debt burden shaping the contextual parameters within which national, urban, community, and household-level social organization is enacted.

External debt impedes the capacity of LDCs to maintain or expand health care delivery to a broad array of the populace as spending on social services becomes increasingly difficult within a context of debt repayment requirements (Bradshaw, Noonan, Gash, & Sershen, 1993; Hill & Pebley, 1989). Further, urban slum prevalence is one expression of the declining capacity of states to provide low-income housing and other basic social services (Davis, 2006; UN-HABITAT, 2003b), a consequence of the down-sizing of public social service efforts in the wake of burgeoning external debt burdens. Debt service payments are a drain on state income that could alternatively be invested in the upgrading of urban public services, and it entrenches export-oriented economic production in order to obtain foreign currency (UN-HABITAT, 2003b). Neoliberal economic policies and stringent structural adjustment conditions attached to development loans, moreover, fuel the social and economic restructuring pushing rural migrants to urban areas ill-equipped to address growing infrastructural demands in the first plane (Davis, 2006; UN-HABITAT, 2003b).

Table 4 highlights the bivariate and partial correlation coefficient calculations between external debt and urban slum prevalence.[8] The top-third of Table 4 illustrates the bivariate correlation. External debt is strongly correlated with urban slum prevalence at a statistically significant level. In turn, more indebted developing countries also exhibit greater urban slum prevalence. The middle-third of Table 4 includes the partial correlation coefficient controlling for GDP per capita. External debt exhibits a moderately strong positive correlation with urban slum prevalence holding constant the influence of economic development. This result is noteworthy as level of economic development in and of itself is argued to be a strong predictor of urban slum prevalence such that more affluent countries per capita are characterized by lower urban slum prevalence (UN-HABITAT, 2003a, 2003b). The bottom-third of Table 4 includes the partial correlation coefficient holding constant GDP per capita and sub-Saharan African countries. The association between debt and urban slum prevalence weakens

Table 4.   External Debt Burden and Urban Slum Prevalence Correlation
Coefficients.

	Urban Slum Prevalence 2001 (%)
Bivariate Correlation Coefficient	
External Debt (% of GNP) 2000	.339***
Partial Correlation Coefficient Controlling for	
GDP Per Capita 2000	
External Debt (% of GNP) 2000	.321***
Partial Correlation Coefficient Controlling for GDP Per Capita	
2000 and Sub-Saharan African Countries ($N = 35$)	
External Debt (% of GNP) 2000	.272**

$^*p < .05$; $^{**}p < .01$; $^{***}p < .001$ (two-tailed tests).

Note: Pearson correlation coefficients are based on the 98 countries listed in Table A1 in the
Appendix. However, data for Namibia and Papua New Guinea were unavailable. Further,
Belarus exhibited a standardized residual beyond three standard deviations on the external debt
variable, raising concerns it constituted an overly influential outlier, and it was omitted from
consideration. The analysis in Table 4, in turn, is based upon the remaining 95 countries. Urban
slum prevalence refers to the percent of the total population living in urban slum conditions in
2001. Data is obtained from UN-HABITAT (2003a). External debt and GDP per capita data
obtained from World Bank (2006b). Consistent with assumptions underlying the statistical
significance tests reported, we performed natural log transformations on those measures with
evidence of non-normal distributions. The following are in natural log form: external debt and
GDP per capita.

but remains statistically significant. This result is notable as it suggests
external debt burden is correlated with urban slum prevalence even after
controlling for sub-Saharan Africa, which generally has the highest
prevalence of slum residents as a proportion of the total population of
any region in the world.

Firebaugh and Beck (1994) dismiss the plausibility of the dependency
theoretical perspective in general and its validity for understanding social
well-being outcomes in the developing countries in particular. They argue

> Recent work in sociology puts forth the revisionist view that foreign dependence, not
> economic growth, is what matters for the poor in LDCs ... This claim of the devastating
> effects of dependence is feckless. Though some types of foreign investment and trade
> may harm LDCs under certain circumstances, robust dependence effects are hard to find
> in the empirical cross-national record. (1994, p. 648)

What Firebaugh and Beck (1994) fail to consider is the remarkable
complexity of cross-national political-economy processes and social well-
being outcomes in the developing countries. Indeed, the robust, deleterious
impact of dependency relations is generally not *direct* but *indirect* through

key intervening factors. For example, in addition to the plausible direct influence upon urban slum conditions, dependency relations have a deleterious effect on economic development (Bradshaw et al., 1993; Chase-Dunn, 1975; London & Williams, 1988; Shen & Williamson, 1997, 1999, 2001; Wimberley & Bello, 1992), fertility rates and therefore population growth (Gallagher, Stokes, & Anderson, 1996; Shen & Williamson, 1999), educational enrollment and attainment levels (Jorgenson, 2004; Jorgenson & Burns, 2004; Shen & Williamson, 1997, 1999, 2001), contraceptive prevalence (Shen & Williamson, 1997, 1999, 2001), organic water pollution (Jorgenson, 2004; Jorgenson & Burns, 2004), and nutritional levels and change (Bradshaw et al., 1993; Wimberley & Bello, 1992) – all factors which act as more proximate and direct predictors of basic indicators of social well-being.

IMPLICATIONS OF URBAN SLUM PREVALENCE FOR POPULATION-LEVEL HEALTH CONCERNS

The determinants of morbidity and mortality are both ultimate or distant and proximate to the event of illness and death (McCarthy & Maine, 1992; Mosley & Chen, 1984). *Distant* determinants include broad socioeconomic factors shaping the context in which individual, household, community, and even national-level social action are enacted. *Proximate* determinants encompass the factors that directly shape morbidity and mortality. Distant determinants often act through more proximate determinants (Mosley & Chen, 1984). However, there is a tendency for social science approaches to focus on the distant determinants, such as income per capita or dependency relations, and then infer the causal mechanisms by which such factors more directly act upon social well-being, leaving the proximate mechanisms an unexplained "black box" (Mosley & Chen, 1984). Conversely, the medical science literature tends to focus on the proximate factors shaping morbidity and mortality but neglects broad, contextual factors (Mosley & Chen, 1984).

Urban slum prevalence arguably constitutes a key intermediate step between broad, socioeconomic determinates and the most proximate factors shaping morbidity and mortality. To establish the connections between distant and proximate factors, to fill-in the "black box" between the social science and medical science perspectives, it may be prudent to include conceptualization of the overstressed and inadequate built urban environment. The context in which people live and die is potentially a powerful mediating influence wherein distant and proximate determinants intersect.

In turn, evidence urban slum prevalence has an impact on population-level measures of social well-being forces consideration of the need for *preventative* in addition to simply *curative* health care efforts in the developing countries. A preventative focus includes evaluation of the underlying social, built, and biophysical environmental factors shaping morbidity and mortality whereas a curative approach emphasizes specific medical interventions employed to combat morbidity as it arises (Ehiri & Prowse, 1999; Hill & Pebley, 1989). A long-standing debate concerns the appropriate policies to pursue within developing countries given the scarce resources available at any given point in time. As Ehiri and Prowse (1999) note, the curative approach has been successful in improving public health in the developing countries, but insufficient consideration of contextual dynamics makes it is difficult to sustain progress over the long term (Ehiri & Prowse, 1999).

Research focused on the social conditions shaping population-level patterns and rates of health and illness remains a promising but contested framework. The wisdom of embracing social factors in addition to a focus on individual-level biological and behavioral risk factors is at times discouraged by more traditional epidemiologists. Zielhuis and Kiemeney (2001) argue the complexities of the medical science and social science approaches pragmatically inhibit meaningful cross-disciplinary research. They suggest

> We therefore believe that epidemiologists, sociologists and psychologists should stick to their field of scientific inquiry ... Stretching borders between epidemiology as a biomedical discipline and sociology only leads to trivial statements, useless for society. (2001, p. 43)

This comment by Zielhuis and Kiemeney is not centered upon the observation that social factors do not shape differential patterns of health and illness but the assertion that there is a general failure to link social dynamics to the "core parameters" of biomedical causation. Researchers have a tendency, in other words, to document the social factors shaping health and illness without embarking on the next logical step, that of drawing inference to the extant body of biomedical research. The critique of Zielhuis and Kiemeney (2001) is noteworthy as it implicitly argues for multifactor and multilevel analysis linking the social and the biological.

Their comment, however, conflates the difficult and the complex with the impossible.

Consistent with the critique by Zielhuis and Kiemeney (2001) more broadly, there is a need for future research efforts that build upon the results of research at variant scales to construct a more comprehensive account of the manner in which broad, social and political-economic dynamics are linked to the core parameters of biomedical causation. We suggest the prevalence of urban slums is a key intervening factor shaped by broad or ultimate determinants but also increasingly the site in which more proximate factors relevant to the extant body of biomedical causation are enacted.

As Cassel (1964) notes, however, the identification of etiologically relevant social dynamics impacting morbidity and mortality should be sensitive to the fact that the factors contributing to the onset of illness may not be the same as those contributing to the lack of recovery from illness. In turn, it is necessary to construct a more comprehensive account of the manner in which urban slum prevalence is a key intervening factor that both promotes greater morbidity and mortality rates as well as a site of concentrated disadvantage wherein access to appropriate health care services is very problematic – in combination with the probable pathways whereby ultimate factors link to more proximate considerations.

It is worth noting, moreover, what may be overlooked by embracing the advice of Zielhuis and Kiemeney (2001) in an uncritical manner; that is, what may be excluded from a broader and deeper "epidemiological discussion" (Macdonald, 2001, p. 47; McPherson, 2001). First, social epidemiology in general and political economy of health theorization in particular promotes a more comprehensive conceptualization of the manner in which political-economic processes and consequent social structural patterns are reflected in recognizable disparities in health and illness. Failure to consider political-economic dynamics only serves to mystify the oppressive socio-organizational relationships that underlie economic production (Singer, 1986).

Second, the built urban environment is in part an expression of cross-national political-economic dynamics and potentially has a substantial influence on the morbidity and mortality rates of marginalized segments of a population that does not equate with the sum of individual-level attributes. An exclusively individual-level approach, moreover, impedes conceptualization of the influence of the built and biophysical environmental factors shaping the challenges to and changes in public health patterns (Gohlke & Portier, 2007). Third, a contextual perspective can highlight "points of leverage" whereby population health patterns can be addressed in a coordinated, concerted manner (Macintyre & Ellaway, 2000, p. 345). Fourth, social epidemiology can contribute to public, democratic debate regarding social patterns of inequality in society and the appropriate policies to pursue in improving public health (Krieger, 2001a). Finally, a focus on the collectivity rather than the individual, as is common in the biomedical model, can correct for class-based biases in diagnosing, treating, and preventing illness (Turshen, 1977).

CONCLUSIONS

Urban social organization can contribute to broad-based social well-being and development but it is also increasingly the site of social, political, and economic marginalization within the developing countries. The contradictory processes of economic globalization call into question the long-standing assumption that urban residents within the developing countries are healthier, better educated, and more prosperous than rural residents as an overarching generalization. The built urban environment in the developing countries is increasingly characterized by substandard living conditions and thereby presents unique public health challenges in general and pressing concerns for children in particular.

Nearly 1 billion people worldwide live in urban slums characterized by lack of access to improved drinking water and sanitation, household overcrowding, lack of durability of residential construction, and insecurity of tenure. The influence of urban slum conditions, moreover, is recognizable in the contradictions that beset urban social organization in the developing countries. In particular, there is increasing evidence of an "urban penalty" wherein urban slum dwellers exhibit poorer health outcomes than non-slum urban residents and even rural residents. Dependency relations enacted among differentially situated countries within the world economy, moreover, is arguably central to the proliferation of urban slum conditions.

Examination of the bivariate and partial correlation coefficients between measures of infant, under-five, and maternal mortality in association with urbanicity and urban slum prevalence, or proportion of the total population living in urban slum conditions, illustrate more urbanized countries exhibit lower mortality levels but countries with greater urban slum conditions are characterized by higher mortality rates. Further, urbanicity has a beneficial positive correlation with measures of life expectancy at birth and gender parity even as urban slum prevalence demonstrates strong negative associations with each. This highlights the increasingly bifurcated composition of urban social organization in the developing countries and supports the assertion of an urban penalty wherein slum residents experience lower levels of social well-being despite the beneficial effects of urbanicity for non-slum urban residents. The deleterious association of urban slum prevalence with measures of social well-being remains strong and statistically significant even after controlling for level of economic development and urban population growth. In turn, the impact of the overstressed and inadequate built urban environment is not synonymous with poverty nor is it a proxy for the rapidity of urban change but constitutes a material, structural pattern fueled by both but exhibiting independent, sui generis properties.

Examination of the 15 overachieving and underachieving LDCs in terms of under-five mortality relative to level of GDP per capita provides evidence the worst performing countries clearly exhibit greater urban slum conditions. The 15 worst performing LDCs have an average urban slum prevalence of 28.4 percent. The 15 best performing countries are characterized by an average of only 5.9 percent. This suggests urban slum prevalence shapes under-five mortality above and beyond the effects of GDP per capita among the best and worst performing countries.

Further, bivariate and partial correlation coefficient calculations demonstrate external debt burden exhibits strong and statistically significant associations with level of urban slum prevalence. This correlation obtains even after controlling for the influence of economic development level. These results are suggestive of the association between dependency dynamics and the form and integrity of urban social organization within the developing countries.

Regression analysis delineating the direct effects of urban slum prevalence on measures of infant, under-five, and maternal mortality as well as gender parity are needed to further disentangle its deleterious influence net alternative predictors identified in the previous research literature. Moreover, few studies from a macro-comparative perspective explicitly focus on the factors shaping urban slum formation.[9] Future research efforts that examine in more detail such concerns would constitute an important contribution to existing knowledge regarding the social production of variant population-level patterns of health and illness indirectly through the promotion of urban slum conditions. Such research efforts are crucial to both acknowledging and articulating the factors driving the urbanization of poverty as embodied in urban slum prevalence and the impact of the built environment on population-level patterns of social well-being in the less developed countries.

NOTES

1. In this chapter "less developed" and "developing" countries refers to non-high income countries (low, lower middle, and upper middle) as categorized by the World Bank (World Bank, 2006a). Reference to "industrialized" and "developed" countries refers to high-income countries.

2. Security of tenure is a recognized aspect of urban slum residence but does not currently constitute a dimension of urban slum measurement at the cross-national level due to insufficient data (see UN-HABITAT, 2003a, pp. 50–51).

3. A growing body of medical science research suggests increasing water *quantity* is as important as improving water *quality* in advancing public health in the developing countries (Cairncross, 2003). The majority of life-threatening diarrheal disease, for example, is not waterborne but transmitted from person to person on hands, food, and through other means within contexts in which there is insufficient water to maintain adequate personal hygiene (Cairncross, 2003).

4. Approximately 94 percent of the global urban slum population resides in the LDCs (UN-HABITAT, 2003a).

5. Note: Figs. 1 and 2 are based on analysis of 165 developing countries as identified by UN-HABITAT (2007b). These countries are listed in Table A1 in the Appendix. Data on annual growth of urban and slum populations are unavailable for Central-Eastern Europe and therefore this category is omitted from Fig. 1.

6. Of note, we define social well-being as consisting of the tangible, measurable non-monetary outcomes of importance to individuals – outcomes enhanced through greater economic and social development. In turn, we define social and gender development as non-monetary considerations that enhance the capacity to engage in purposive social action oriented towards improving social well-being and economic development.

7. Consistent with normative practice in quantitative, macro-comparative research, the developing countries under examination in Tables 2–4 are restricted to non-high income countries, as defined by the World Bank (2006a) for 2000, and those with a minimum population of 1 million to avoid anomalies related to low population countries. This produces a database of 98 countries, listed in Table A1 in the Appendix. Infant and under-five mortality refer to the probability of death expressed per 1,000 live births. The life expectancy at birth measure is an estimate of the number of years a newborn child would live if subject to the mortality risks prevailing for their cross-section of the population at the time of their birth. For more information on the infant, under-five, and life expectancy measures see UNICEF (2007). Maternal mortality refers to the adjusted figure which is intended to compensate for the widespread underreporting of maternal deaths by national authorities and expresses the annual number of deaths from pregnancy related causes during pregnancy or within 42 days of the termination of a pregnancy per 100,000 live births. For more information see World Health Organization (WHO) (2007).

8. External debt consists of the sum of short-term external debt plus total debt service payments due over the life of existing loans expressed as a percent of gross national product (GNP).

9. Previous research from a macro-comparative perspective does examine overurbanization (see Bradshaw, 1985; Timberlake & Kentor, 1983). Overurbanization

refers to levels of urbanization determined to be excessive relative to a given level of GDP per capita, suggesting urban agglomeration without parallel economic development. This is very different, however, from the examination of urban slum prevalence, which is arguably a more appropriate measure of the influence of the built environment. Of note, Bradshaw et al. (1993) examine the impact of overurbanization on under-five mortality within LDCs. Their results do not illustrate overurbanization has a statistically significant direct effect on child mortality.

REFERENCES

Agarwal, S., & Taneja, S. (2005). All slums are not equal: Child health conditions among the urban poor. *Indian Pediatrics, 42*, 233–244.

Amin, S. (1974). *Accumulation on a world scale*. New York: Monthly Review Press.

Awasthi, S., & Agarwal, S. (2003). Determinants of childhood mortality and morbidity in urban slums in India. *Indian Pediatrics, 40*, 1145–1161.

Bartlett, S. (2003). Water, sanitation, and urban children: The need to go beyond 'Improved' provision. *Environment and Urbanization, 15*(2), 57–70.

Bolay, J.-C. (2006). Slums and urban development: Questions on society and globalization. *The European Journal of Development Research, 18*(2), 284–298.

Bradshaw, Y. W. (1985). Overurbanization and underdevelopment in sub-Saharan Africa: A cross-national study. *Studies in Comparative International Development, 20*(3), 74–101.

Bradshaw, Y. W., Noonan, R., Gash, L., & Sershen, C. B. (1993). Borrowing against the future: Children and third world indebtedness. *Social Forces, 71*(3), 629–656.

Brown, V. J. (2003). Give me shelter: The global housing crisis. *Environmental Health Perspectives, 111*(2), A92–A99.

Cairncross, S. (2003). Water supply and sanitation: Some misconceptions. *Tropical Medicine and International Health, 8*(3), 193–195.

Caldwell, J. C. (1990). Cultural and social factors influencing mortality levels in developing countries. *The ANNALS of the American Academy of Political and Social Science, 510*(1), 44–59.

Cassel, J. (1964). Social science theory as a source of hypotheses in epidemiological research. *American Journal of Public Health, 54*(9), 1482–1488.

Chase-Dunn, C. (1975). The effects of international economic dependence on development and inequality: A cross-national study. *American Sociological Review, 40*, 720–738.

Chase-Dunn, C. (1989). *Global formation: Structures of the world-economy*. Cambridge, MA: Blackwell Publishers.

Davis, M. (2006). *Planet of slums*. New York: Verso.

Ehiri, J. E., & Prowse, J. M. (1999). Child health promotion in developing countries: The case for integration of environmental and social interventions? *Health Policy and Planning, 14*(1), 1–10.

Elling, R. H. (1981). The capitalist world-system and international health. *International Journal of Health Services, 11*(1), 21–51.

Engels, F. (1968[1845]). *The condition of the working class in England*. W. O. Henderson & W. H. Chaloner (Eds & Trans.). Stanford, CA: Stanford University Press.

Fernandez, A., Mondkar, J., & Mathai, S. (2003). Urban slum-specific issues in neonatal survival. *Indian Pediatrics, 40,* 1161–1166.

Firebaugh, G., & Beck, F. D. (1994). Does economic growth benefit the masses? Growth, dependence, and welfare in the third world. *American Sociological Review, 59,* 631–653.

Frank, A. G. (1966). The development of underdevelopment. *Monthly Review, 18*(7), 17–31.

Gallagher, S. K., Stokes, R. G., & Anderson, A. B. (1996). Economic disarticulation and fertility in less developed nations. *The Sociological Quarterly, 37*(2), 227–244.

Ghosh, S., & Shah, D. (2004). Nutritional problems in urban slum children. *Indian Pediatrics, 41,* 682–696.

Gohlke, J. M., & Portier, C. J. (2007). The forest for the trees: A systems approach to human health research. *Environmental Health Perspectives, 115*(9), 1261–1263.

Hill, K., & Pebley, A. R. (1989). Child mortality in the developing world. *Population and Development Review, 15*(4), 657–687.

Jorgenson, A. K. (2004). Global inequality, water pollution, and infant mortality. *The Social Science Journal, 41,* 279–288.

Jorgenson, A. K., & Burns, T. J. (2004). Globalization, the environment, and infant mortality: A cross-national study. *Humboldt Journal of Social Relations, 28*(1), 7–52.

Krieger, N. (1999). Embodying inequality: A review of concepts, measures, and methods for studying health consequences of discrimination. *International Journal of Health Services, 29*(2), 295–352.

Krieger, N. (2001a). Historical roots of social epidemiology: Socioeconomic gradients in health and contextual analysis. *International Journal of Epidemiology, 30,* 899–900.

Krieger, N. (2001b). Theories for social epidemiology in the 21st century: An ecosocial perspective. *International Journal of Epidemiology, 30*(4), 668–677.

Link, B. G., & Phelan, J. C. (1995). Social conditions as fundamental causes of disease. *Journal of Health and Social Behavior, 35*(Extra Issue), 80–94.

Link, B. G., & Phelan, J. C. (1996). Understanding sociodemographic differences in health: The role of fundamental social causes. *American Journal of Public Health, 86*(4), 471–473.

London, B., & Williams, B. A. (1988). Multinational corporate penetration, protest, and basic needs provision in non-core nations: A cross-national analysis. *Social Forces, 66*(3), 747–773.

Macdonald, K. I. (2001). Social epidemiology. A way? *International Journal of Epidemiology, 30,* 46–47.

Macintyre, S., & Ellaway, A. (2000). Ecological approaches: Rediscovering the role of the physical and social environment. In: L. F. Berkman & I. Kawachi (Eds), *Social epidemiology* (pp. 332–348). New York: Oxford University Press.

McCarthy, J., & Maine, D. (1992). A framework for analyzing the determinants of maternal mortality. *Studies in Family Planning, 23*(1), 23–33.

McKinlay, J. B. (1981). A case for refocusing upstream: The political economy of illness. In: P. Conrad & R. Kern (Eds), *The sociology of health and illness: Critical perspectives* (pp. 613–633). New York: St. Martin's Press.

McPherson, K. (2001). Epidemiology? Keep it broad and deep. *International Journal of Epidemiology, 30,* 48.

Mogford, L. (2004). Structural determinants of child mortality in sub-Saharan Africa: A cross-national study of economic and social influences from 1970–1997. *Social Biology, 51*(3/4), 94–120.

Morgan, L. M. (1987). Dependency theory in the political economy of health: An anthropological critique. *Medical Anthropology Quarterly, 1*(2), 131–154.

Mosley, W. H., & Chen, L. C. (1984). An analytical framework for the study of child survival in developing countries. *Population and Development Review, 10*(Suppl.), 25–45.

Satterthwaite, D. (1993). The impact on health of urban environments. *Environment and Urbanization, 5*(2), 87–111.

Scanlan, S. J. (2004). Women, food security, and development in less-industrialized societies: Contributions and challenges for the new century. *World Development, 32*(11), 1807–1829.

Sclar, E., Garau, P., & Carolini, G. (2005). The 21st century health challenge of slums and cities. *The Lancet, 365*(March 5), 901–903.

Shen, C., & Williamson, J. B. (1997). Child mortality, women's status, economic dependency, and state strength: A cross-national study of less developed countries. *Social Forces, 76*(2), 667–694.

Shen, C., & Williamson, J. B. (1999). Maternal mortality, women's status, and economic dependency in less developed countries: A cross-national analysis. *Social Science and Medicine, 49*, 197–214.

Shen, C., & Williamson, J. B. (2001). Accounting for cross-national differences in infant mortality decline (1965–1991) among less developed countries: Effects of women's status, economic dependency, and state strength. *Social Indicators Research, 53*, 257–288.

Singer, M. (1986). Developing a critical perspective in medical anthropology. *Medical Anthropology Quarterly, 17*(5), 128–129.

Timberlake, M., & Kentor, J. (1983). Economic dependence, overurbanization, and economic growth: A study of less developed countries. *The Sociological Quarterly, 24*, 489–507.

Turshen, M. (1977). The political ecology of disease. *Review of Radical Political Economics, 9*(1), 45–60.

United Nations Children's Fund (UNICEF). (2007). *The state of the world's children.* New York: United Nations.

United Nations Development Programme (UNDP). (2006). *Human Development Report 2006. Beyond Scarcity: Power, Poverty, and the Global Water Crisis.* NY: United Nations.

United Nations Human Settlements Programme (UN-HABITAT). (2003a). *Slums of the World: The face of urban poverty in the new millennium?* London: Earthscan. Available at www.unhabitat.org

United Nations Human Settlements Programme (UN-HABITAT). (2003b). *The challenge of slums: Global report on human settlements 2003.* London: Earthscan. Available at www.unhabitat.org

United Nations Human Settlements Programme (UN-HABITAT). (2006). *State of the world's cities report 2006/7.* London: Earthscan. Available at www.unhabitat.org

United Nations Human Settlements Programme (UN-HABITAT). (2007a). *Slums: some definitions.* Available at www.unhabitat.org, accessed May, 2007.

United Nations Human Settlements Programme (UN-HABITAT). (2007b). *Slum estimate data.* Available at ww2.unhabitat.org/programmes/guo/statistics.asp, accessed May, 2007.

United Nations Human Settlements Programme (UN-HABITAT). (2007c). *The urban penalty: The poor die young.* Available at www.unhabitat.org, accessed May, 2007.

Vlahov, D., Freudenberg, N., Proietti, F., Ompad, D., Quinn, A., Nandi, V., & Galea, S. (2007). Urban as a determinant of health. *Journal of Urban Health: Bulletin of the New York Academy of Medicine, 84*(1), i16–i26.

Wagstaff, A., Bustreo, F., Bryce, J., & Claeson, M. (2004). Child health: Reaching the poor. *American Journal of Public Health, 94*(5), 726–736.

Waitzkin, H. (1981). The social origins of illness: A neglected history. *International Journal of Health Services, 11*(1), 77–103.

Wallerstein, I. (1974). *The modern world system I: Capitalist agriculture and the origins of the European world-economy in the sixteenth century.* New York: Academic Press.

Wickrama, K. A. S., & Lorenz, F. O. (2002). Women's status, fertility decline, and women's health in developing countries: Direct and indirect influences of social status on health. *Rural Sociology, 67*(2), 255–277.

Wimberley, D. W., & Bello, R. (1992). Effects of foreign investment, exports, and economic growth on third world food consumption. *Social Forces, 70*(4), 895–921.

World Bank. (2005). *World development Indicators.* Washington, DC: World Bank.

World Bank. (2006a). *Historical income classifications.* Retrieved October, 2006 (http://www.worldbank.org). Washington, DC: World Bank.

World Bank. (2006b). *2006 world development indicators online.* Washington, DC: The World Bank. Available at http://www.worldbank.org

World Health Organization (WHO). (2007). *Maternal mortality in 2005: Estimates developed by WHO, UNICEF, UNFPA, and the World Bank.* Geneva, Switzerland: World Health Organization. Available at www.who.org

Zielhuis, G. A., & Kiemeney, L. A. L. M. (2001). Social epidemiology? No way. *International Journal of Epidemiology, 30*, 43–44.

APPENDIX

Table A1. Less Developed Countries Included in the Analyses.

Eastern Asia
China
Hong Kong*
Macao*
Korea, North*
Korea, South*
Mongolia

South-Eastern Asia
Brunei*
Cambodia
Indonesia
Laos
Malaysia
Myanmar*
Philippines
Thailand
Timor-Leste*
Vietnam

Western Asia
Armenia
Azerbaijan
Bahrain*
Georgia*
Iraq*
Israel*
Jordan
Kuwait*
Lebanon
Palestinian Territory*
Oman*
Qatar*
Saudi Arabia*
Syria
Turkey
United Arab Emirates*
Yemen

Southern Asia
Afghanistan*
Bangladesh

Bhutan*
India
Iran
Kazakhstan
Kyrgyzstan
Nepal
Pakistan
Sri Lanka
Tajikistan
Turkmenistan*
Uzbekistan

Sub-Saharan Africa
Angola
Benin
Botswana
Burkina Faso
Burundi
Cameroon
Cape Verde*
Central African Repub.*
Chad
Comoros*
Congo
Congo, Dem. Republic*
Côte d'Ivoire
Equatorial Guinea*
Eritrea
Ethiopia
Gabon
Gambia
Ghana
Guinea
Guinea-Bissau
Kenya
Lesotho
Liberia*
Madagascar
Malawi
Mali
Mauritania

Mozambique
Namibia
Niger
Nigeria
Rwanda
Saint Helena*
Sao Tome and Principe*
Senegal
Seychelles*
Sierra Leone
Somalia*
South Africa
Sudan
Tanzania
Togo
Uganda
Zambia
Zimbabwe

Northern Africa
Algeria
Egypt*
Libya*
Morocco
Tunisia
Western Sahara*

Latin America-Caribbean
Anguilla*
Antigua and Barbuda*
Argentina
Aruba*
Bahamas*
Barbados*
Belize*
Bermuda*
Bolivia
Brazil
British Virgin Islands*
Cayman Islands*
Chile

Table A1.   *(Continued).*

Colombia	Montserrat*	*Eastern Europe*
Costa Rica	Netherlands Antilles*	Albania
Cuba*	Nicaragua	Belarus
Dominica*	Panama	Bulgaria
Dominican Republic	Paraguay	Croatia
Ecuador*	Peru	Czech Republic
El Salvador	Puerto Rico*	Estonia
Falkland Islands*	Saint Kitts and Nevis*	Hungary
French Guiana*	Saint Lucia*	Latvia
Greenland*	St. Vincent-Grenadines*	Lithuania*
Grenada*	Saint-Pierre-et-Miq.*	Macedonia*
Guadeloupe*	Suriname*	Moldova
Guatemala	Trinidad and Tobago	Poland*
Guyana*	Turks and Caicos*	Romania
Haiti*	Uruguay	Russia
Honduras	U.S. Virgin Islands*	Serbia and Montenegro*
Jamaica	Venezuela	Slovakia
Martinique*		Ukraine
Mexico	*Oceania*	
	Papua New Guinea	

Note: * Indicates countries included in the analyses illustrated in Figs. 1 and 2 ($N = 165$) but omitted from analyses highlighted in Tables 2–4. All non-designated countries are included in the analyses illustrated in Tables 2–4 ($N = 98$). Regional classification is based on United Nations Statistics Division standards.

UNSETTLED BORDERS OF CARE: MEDICAL TOURISM AS A NEW DIMENSION IN AMERICA'S HEALTH CARE CRISIS

Elizabeth Anne Jenner

ABSTRACT

Health care has become one of the paramount issues of the 21st century as governments and individuals grapple the complex problems associated with contemporary medical care such as cost, affordability, and shifting demographic trends. One response has been the growth of medical tourism (sometimes called health tourism or global healthcare). Medical tourism is an example of how the forces of globalization are re-shaping what has previously been a relatively stable localized service, medical treatment, in the face of changes to health care. While traveling to distant locations in search of health restoring locations is not new as the affluent have long traveled to spas or exotic locales to derive health benefits. What has changed is who is doing it and why they are doing it as insurers and patients alike become eager participants in the outsourcing of medical care. The rising number of uninsured and underinsured Americans, particularly in the middle class, has been coupled with effective marketing by medical tourism companies to produce growing numbers of Americans

Care for Major Health Problems and Population Health Concerns:
Impacts on Patients, Providers and Policy
Research in the Sociology of Health Care, Volume 26, 235–249
Copyright © 2008 by Emerald Group Publishing Limited
All rights of reproduction in any form reserved
ISSN: 0275-4959/doi:10.1016/S0275-4959(08)26011-4

traveling to foreign countries for healthcare. China, India, Korea, Malaysia, the Philippines, South Africa, and Thailand are only a few of the competitors for overseas patients as a source for economic development. Using analytic frameworks of Immanuel Wallerstein and Anthony Giddens to provide a social analysis of this phenomenon yields an exploration of this trend.

Health care in the United States has been gaining greater social and political importance in public debates about how best to provide health care for 300 million Americans amid increasing costs and changing demographics. These debates have become steadily more intense as workers (both union and non-union workers) politicians, policy makers, employers, and others try to figure out how to provide and fund health care services (Milstein & Smith, 2007; Smith, 2004; El Taguri, 2007). The steady decline in the number of U.S. employers providing medical insurance has added to the pressures felt by American health care consumers (Blumenthal, 2006; Fuchs & Ezekiel, 2005). In response, a growing number patients have begun seeking medical care outside of the customary healthcare structure and are now looking to the international community for medical treatment. International travel, especially to destinations in developing nations, is now easier, faster, and less expensive than in previous generations and as a result patients are more likely to take advantage of medical treatment offered abroad. Additionally, the advent of international trade agreements such as General Agreement on Trade in Services (GATS) the healthcare destinations available to today's medical consumers are considerably wider. For some, this has taken the form of medical tourism, the latest impetus in the ongoing process of globalization.

Medical tourism differs from health tourism in that medical tourists seek specific medical treatment rather than a health-promoting trip to a resort, spa, or fitness facility. While there is no clear consensus on its meaning, generally medical tourism is understood to be the blending of tourism and medical treatment for both elective and necessary surgical and medical procedure(s), as well as for dental procedure(s). Changing dynamics within economic structures and relationships have created both opportunities and challenges in the delivery of health care requiring new approaches to solving old problems. Observers maintain that forces that have given other forms of globalization (technology, mobility, and the flow of capital) are facilitating the globalization process in medical care (Smith, 2004). The ongoing globalization of health care is a rising trend evident in the increase in medical tourism,[1] especially internationally.

The phenomenon of medical, or health tourism, dates back to at least to the ancient Greeks as they traveled to distant destinations to improve or restore their health. Virtually every society has engaged in some form of medical tourism and the US is no exception. Medical tourism has been a trend in American medicine for nearly two hundred years; however, recently the numbers, flow, and direction of medical tourists has begun to change Centers for Disease Control. In the past, patients in the United States have practiced medical tourism within national boundaries with only a small percentage of patients traveling outside national borders. Until recently, the main flow of patients across United States borders has, been in rather than out, of the country. Medical clinics and hospitals in Western Europe and the United States have targeted affluent international travelers seeking the very best in medical treatment since the late 19th century. American medicine was firmly established as the locus of medical innovation and quality during the post-World War II era with the development of an arsenal of medications to treat a wide range of illnesses such as diabetes, arthritis, and infections as well as the advent of successful childhood vaccines.

This trend continued and expanded during the 1960s as affluent patients journeyed to the United States in search of clinical, technological, and innovative medical facilities that produced remarkable health outcomes and breakthroughs. During this period the United States boasted unrivaled medical facilities and funds to fuel research and innovation in many aspects of medical treatment (Starr, 1984). The well-publicized "miracles of modern medicine" of this era helped to fuel the steady rise in international patients drawn to the United States or treatment. In the late 1980s, renowned US medical research centers, like the Mayo Clinic, Stanford University Medical Center, Johns Hopkins Hospital, and Cleveland Clinic, established formal programs to attract foreign patients. These programs provided services like interpreters, assistance with visa and travel, plus VIP travel and accommodation amenities including suites and specially designated luxury facilities. By the end of the 20th century, approximately a quarter of a million international patients were seeking medical treatment in the United States annually. Yet, this flow of patients has become more complex as Americans travel overseas to developing nations for medical treatment creating a more significant cross current of patients moving across borders.

As stated earlier, health care has been a topic for discussion and debate for many years but recently this discussion has taken on a new intensity and a more global theme. The reasons for this are the pressures, both exogenous and endogenous, on the delivery of medical care. An example of the complex interplay of these forces is evident; in attempts by developing nations to restructure their health care options they looked at models of health care delivery in other countries, most notably the United States and Canada. A significant number of physicians from developing nations trained, and acquired skills from their training in the United States and Western Europe that they brought back to their country of origin causing an increase in sub-specialty expertise and technical abilities. As a consequence medical centers and hospitals in developing countries are now able to attract patients from Western Europe, Canada, and the US as a new revenue source for economic development.

> That patients from abroad would become a source for economic development in the developing world is explicable within the broad context of the transformative nature of globalization. Maciel (2003) contends "the dynamic relations activated by this revolution [globalization] thrust on the stage previously unknown social actors and issues; they redefine some of the traditional ones; they displace or destroy many others". (p. 42)

It has also led to the development of transnational alliances specifically directed toward increasing this new patient base and revenue source. Health care, especially the Western or American model of health care, is a commodity (not simply a necessary service) that is marketed to international travelers and those who are in a social class that can afford it.

While it is quite difficult to get precise cost estimates on even the most common medical/surgical procedures there are some indicators of the cost savings possible through medical tourism. Table 1 illustrates some of the cost differences between the US, India, and Thailand for several common procedures and the cost difference is striking for all procedures. For example, the most expensive procedure, a coronary bypass graft, is 12–15% of the average cost of this procedure at US facilities. Even for patients with the standard 20% co-pay insurance their out-of-pocket costs for this procedure would exceed the cost of the procedure in either India or Thailand. Since abdominoplasty (tummy tuck) is an elective procedure (not medically necessary) the patient would typically be required to pay 100% of the costs if done in the United States. The cost associated with this procedure alone would be 50–70% higher than what it would cost if done India or Thailand.

The financial savings possible through medical tourism is luring patients and insurers alike. A cursory comparison between the procedure costs listed in Table 1 for procedures obtained in developing countries reveals significantly lower costs and seem very attractive to US patients with high co-payments and deductibles medical insurance plans, those with no medical

Table 1. Cost Comparisons of Selected Procedures by Country.

Procedure Costs is US dollars[a,b,c]	USA	India	Thailand
Total Hip replacement	3,500–4,000	4,150	5,600
Cardiac Angiography	19,475	480	1,100
Cardiac Angioplasty	41,810	3,500	8,575
Coronary Artery Bypass	81,600	9,500	12,650
Breast Augmentation	8,750	2,075	2,725
Abdominoplasty	8,000	2,700	4,276

[a]These costs are an average the data retrieved on April 19, 2008 from the following four websites: Medical Tourism Partners Inc., http://www.medicaltourismpartners.com/index.php?link = medical; the Bair and Helft Consulting Group, http://www.bairandhelft.com/BH_Projects.html; Healthbase, http://www.healthbase.com/; and U.S. Agency for Healthcare Research and Quality, http://www.hcup-us.ahrq.gov/reports/methods.jsp all accessed April 18, 2008.
[b]Not all cases had data; some estimates include only two data points.
[c]Cost estimates of any medical procedures performed in the US are extremely difficult to obtain from the providers. The above estimates rely on data sources listed above.

insurance, or those seeking elective procedures not covered by medical insurance. With possible cost savings of between 80% and 90% on many of the most common medical procedures, medical insurers have begun to take notice. Some insurers are beginning to taking advantage of the lowered costs by paying for medical services obtained from foreign providers. One example of this new practice is Blue Shield of California's *Access Baja* (Access Baja BlueShield, 2008). This plan option permits Blue Shield customers to receive coverage for procedures and treatments in Mexico at authorized clinics and physicians. In addition, Blue Cross Blue Shield of South Carolina has included Bumrungrad International Hospital (located in Thailand) in its network of authorized providers. Both of these insurers are example of companies taking advantage of the lowered costs and commensurate saving by seeking medical care beyond the United States border. Currently, the majority of US medical insurers do not currently cover medical expenses, except necessary emergency medical care, incurred by patients as a result of seeking treatment in foreign countries. Given the potential savings to insurers and patients alike, it is reasonable to expect that this will change in the near future as employers seek innovative means of controlling health care costs. Employers and patients are turning to a new and growing number of medical tour providers like Medical Tourism Partners (MTP), One World Healthcare, MedTrava, Healthbase, and MedRetreat among others.

Through medical tourism companies, international travelers can purchase access to western style medical clinics in India, Thailand, Jordan, Argentina, Singapore, and other distant locations. These organizations represent the newest entrepreneurial entrants in the global delivery of patients to overseas health care providers while providing medical options for consumers. Companies that specialize in medical tourism market a full range of services to their customers that typically includes interpreters, complete pricing and costs for any medical procedures up-front, lists of specialists complete with credentials, lists of accredited treatment facilities, and a trip coordinator. The burgeoning medical tourism industry and companies that specialize in medical tourism serve to deepen the globalization of health care. Moreover, these companies are marketing medical tourism almost exclusively towards middle-class Americans. The target market are those who are under-insured, uninsured, have large deductibles, or want (or need) services or treatment(s) that they must pay for out of pocket, and treatments not yet approved in the United States. While there is no specific data on the number of patients' worldwide who contribute to the rise in medical tourism there are government figures from India, Thailand, and Jordan among others that indicate it is on the rise and becoming a worldwide multi-billion dollar industry (Mutchnick, Stern, & Moyer, 2005; Turner, 2007). Some estimates are that although about 500,000–750,00 patients traveled from the United States seeking care in the developing world this number will increase to over 1 million in the next 2 years. With an estimated 46–47 million American lacking health insurance and 120 million lacking dental insurance it is possible that the number of patients seeking medical care abroad is far too conservative.

As medical tourism and medical tourism companies move into public awareness and debates about health care, it is reasonable to conclude that utilization of medical care services in developing countries will continue to climb. Indeed Kher (2006) contends that medical tourism may have "the potential of doing to the US health-care system what the Japanese auto industry did to American carmakers" (p. 44). The capability of medical tourism to transform the health care industry sparked enough Congressional interest to warrant a hearing into the issue. The United States Senate, Special Committee on Aging, held Hearings[2] in June 2006 on the subject of medical tourism as a way to control health costs. During these hearings the Committee heard from industry experts, physicians, and patients about the impact medical tourism may have on the American health care system (United States Senate Special Committee on Aging, 2006, pp. 3–4). In addition, potential risks associated with medical tourism received attention.

Some of the possible hazards discussed were poor quality of medical care, poor follow-up on treatment once they return to the United States, unfamiliar language, and weak or non-existent consumer protection laws (United States Senate Special Committee on Aging, 2006). The Hearings resulted in a call for a task force to explore the overall impact, costs, and patient safety of medical care obtained out of the country. The testimony revealed that despite the potential risks of seeking medical care abroad patients and employers are beginning to see medical tourism as a new and viable option to help reduce health care costs. The lure of cost saving for purchasers and patient is one aspect of the growth in medical tourism as is the changing economic structure in many developing nations.

The international market for services has also been fueled by recent moves to privatize health care in several of the former socialist countries and democratic countries with national health care (Mutchnick et al., 2005; Skarbinski et al., 2002). This move has further fueled a consumerism of medical services and technologies (Duffy, 1997; Fineberg, 1995; Gómez-Dantés & Frenk, 1995). The governments of many countries are actively pursuing medical tourism as a new source of economic development and to obtain a share of this billion-dollar industry. Some have established offices specifically designed to promote and increase medical tourism to their countries. Some of the countries that are actively involved in promoting medical tourism are Costa Rica, Cuba, India, Thailand, Hungary, Israel, Jordan, Lithuania, and the Philippines (MacIntosh, 2004). In addition, U.S. Commercial Service, an entity within the U.S. Department of Commerce, states, "the growth of medical tourism in the Philippines offers many good opportunities for U.S. sellers of medical equipment and instruments" (U.S. Commercial Service, 2008). Just as the emergence of for-profit hospitals changed the landscape of US health care so too will worldwide medical tourism (Starr, 1984). As the demand for medical treatment and desperation in some cases to obtain treatments unavailable or unaffordable in their resident country consumers are reshaping the delivery of health care on a global scale. Just as consumerism had transformed other aspects of the global economy so too are medical consumers. Duffy asserts that

> Conventional wisdom would argue that there are two pre-requisites for consumerism: a public that is able to express its interests and preferences, and a willingness of provider of goods and services to deliver the products that consumer's desire. (Duffy, 1997, p. 301)

The drive to provide medical services health care consumers want has opened the door for services provided by medical tourism companies. These new health care corporations are moving into, and shaping, a global market for health care and medical treatment. The globalization of health care represents a shift from community based health care providers and hospitals, which delivered health care for the local population, to a progressively more global system. Health care is transforming into a system controlled by large mega health care corporations, consumer demand, employers, governmental offices of economic development, and increasingly insurers. The decentralization of capital, which has happened in industry after industry, is often closely linked to the internationalization of industries (Burbach, 2001). An example of this trend is the increased use of telemedicine as an accepted means of patient treatment and interaction. This is a recent development in health care delivery that moves medical treatment physically away from the patient though the use of the Internet, telecommunications, video, and email (Sinha, 2000). Support for telemedicine is growing in the face of economic restructuring in health care and burgeoning costs. For example, a significant number of digitally recorded diagnostic images, like X-rays, are transmitted to another country for interpretation. Some US patients consult their physicians via email, and receive diagnosis and treatment via email in return. These e-visits are billed to the patient and are being covered and paid for by insurance. Health care is becoming increasingly impersonal and technologically dispensed developments that facilitate the growth of globalization of health care.

Since a central component of this assertion is the phenomena of "globalization" as it relates to health care, it is necessary to develop an understanding of what this means in the context of medical care. Globalization often understood as an economic phenomenon in which raw materials, goods and services are purchased and sold on a world market rather than a national or local one. Robertson (1992) contends that there is a broader view and description of globalization; "globalization as a concept refers both to the compression of the world and intensification of consciousness of the world as a whole ... both concrete global interdependence and consciousness of the global whole in the twentieth century" (p. 8). This is a useful conceptualization of globalization[3] for the purposes of understanding health care in an era of ever deteriorating national, technological, mental and physical boundaries in the delivery of health care services.

There are several ways to make sense of the ways globalization is transforming health care. "Globalization is not occurring in a vacuum ... Receding government, deregulation, and the shrinking of social obligations are the domestic counterparts of the intertwining of national economies" (Rodrik, 1997, p. 85). Shifting health care options illustrate the increasingly global nature of health care and point to the importance of a worldwide perspective to appreciate the contemporary transformation of health care and its broad global implications.

Health care globalization manifests itself in several ways (some have already been discussed) and central to all of these is standardization of medical knowledge and practices to meet the consumer demands and expectations of medical tourists from the United States, Canada, and Western Europe. Health care globalization includes the "exchange of ideas about medical science, particularly the scientific canon, as well as about technological progress in medical innovations, ... [which] easily cross borders" (Björkman & Altenstetter, 1997, p. 9).

Anthony Giddens (1990) describes globalization as

The intensification of worldwide social relations which link distant locations in such a way that local happenings are shaped by events occurring many miles away and vice versa. This is a dialectic process because such local happenings may move in an obverse direction from the very distanciated relations that shape them. Local transformation is as much a part of globalization as the lateral extension of the social connections across time and space. (p. 64)

This view seems to be reinforced by the practical dialogue about health care changes, health care policy reform, and emerging trends in the provision of care. There are globalizing pressures on the health care dialectic process that can be discussed by globalization theory. Giddens (1990) asserts "one aspect of the dialectical nature of globalization is the push and pull between tendencies inherent in the reflexivity of the system of states on the one hand, and the sovereignty of particular states on the other" (p. 73). This assertion implies a reciprocity of power and agency in the transformative, globalizing dialectic process at both the local and global levels.

Giddens' (1990) focus on the locality of transformation as an integral part of globalization can help explain why local systems of health care are both necessary for, and susceptible to, globalization. He asserts that "locales are thoroughly penetrated by and shaped in terms of social influences quite distant from them ... the 'visible form' of the locale conceals the distanciated relations which determine its nature" (Giddens, 1990, p. 19). The idea that global forces affect local health care has been part of the ongoing dialogue within the health care policy debate about the health care. Indeed it has been pointed out "health is affected by economic, political, technological, and cultural transformations" (Gómez-Dantés & Frenk, 1995, p. 13). Presumably this statement reflects the uneven and inter-connected nature of health care delivery on a global scale. Giddens is useful in understanding the changes that are taking place in health care. In addition, Giddens (1990) statement that globalization "is a process of uneven development that fragments as it coordinates" (p. 175) seems remarkably apropos to the case of health care given the increased reliance on medical specialties in the last quarter century.

Gidden's (1990) analysis of globalization does not address the interlocking and interdependent nature of the economic organization of the health care industry and the political institutions of nation states. Björkman and Altenstetter (1997) argue that the process of globalizing health care can be traced to the early days of colonialism. This argument exposes a significant problem in applying Giddens' globalization theory to the changing contours of health care delivery because he contends that globalization can only occur where economic and social structures are mutually insulated from each other. The idea of the 'dialectic' nature of globalization Giddens (1990) borrows heavily from Marx while rejecting Marx's emphasis on economics and social class as factors in social change. However, the state's interest in the provision and consumption of health care services do not exist separately from its political and economic structure. Giddens' globalization analysis is not the only theory that can be used to examine the evolving global nature of health care and medical tourism.

World-system model of analysis developed by Immanuel Wallerstein (1974) provides a systematic analysis of what would otherwise seem to be disparate and unrelated events. The rise of medical tourism can be seen as more than the individual agency of social actors (patients, politicians, and health care providers). Using a world-system framework it can be argued that the structural pressures and changes to health care delivery are really part of a single economic stream of global expansion of capitalism across geographic boundaries. Wallerstein (1974) asserts the capitalist world-economy has expanded the geographic boundaries of the capitalist system as a whole; when applied to the current globalization of health care this argument carries a significance regarding the globalization of medical care and medical tourism as a facet of capitalist expansion. Certainly the expansion of US-based health care into other countries can be seen as reminiscent of the kind of core periphery capitalist expansion that he describes in his world-systems analysis. This feature of Wallerstein's analysis is useful in tracing the global development of health care service providers, again especially in the case of the for-profit health care providers that are central to the growing medical tourism industry.

In his analysis, Wallerstein pays particular attention to the emergence and development of a unified world market, and the concomitant international division of labor. This could be a key framework from which to see the globalizing of health care as capitalism's continued expansion through medical tourism. Wallerstein's argument of the exploitation of the periphery by the core can be applied to the globalization of health care, if we define US medicine as part of the core[5] and the new privatized health care market as periphery. Within this framework the role of health care professionals would be that of the semi-periphery. Further, Wallerstein has defined a world-system, as one in which there is an extensive division of labor. This division of labor is not simply a functional one based on occupational segmentation but is also geographical segmentation, which perpetuates economic inequality between core and periphery. This seems especially true regarding the division of labor in medical tourism that relies on the lower wages of workers in the developing world.

Understanding the division of labor allows us to see how the ranges of economic tasks, which are not evenly distributed throughout the world-system, are an integral part of the capitalist expansion of health care. For the most part, the segmentation of economic tasks is a function of the social organization of work, one that magnifies and legitimizes the ability of some groups within the system to exploit the labor of others. Medical tourism companies are an example of a calculated exploitation in order to build wealth for 'core' capitalist economies.

In addition to the wage differences that this creates there is also a difference in access to health care. Those in the elite social classes have a broader range of health care choices than those in the lower economic segments of any society. Even employees with health care provided through employers are facing a negative change in their access to health care (Blumenthal, 2006; Fuchs & Ezekiel, 2005). One facet of this is "the use of managed care [in a 'free market'] is that financial as well as organizational incentives now favor the under provision rather than the over provision of services" (Rodwin, 1997, p. 48). In the early 1990s managed care heath insurance program were able to control costs by the use of strict utilization review and gatekeeper prior authorization (Gabel et al., 2005). However, these techniques of success served to fuel the consumer backlash against managed care that began in 2000 resulting in a slacking of stringent oversight by insurer. Those who are able to gain access to the increasingly expensive or limited services are more likely to be able to move outside the state or employer sponsored health care services and purchase them directly. An example of this is the practice of Canadian patients traveling to the United States to receive health care that they pay for out of their own pocket. This practice has also occurred under Socialist medicine programs as those with resources and the ability to travel to Western Europe for medical care did (Duffy, 1997). The latest shifts in the flow of patients from industrialized countries to developing nations may signal a new expansion of the world economy that continues the exploitation of the periphery or developing nations of the world economy.

Wallerstein (1974) insists that looking at the "distinction between a peripheral area of a given world-economy and the external arena of the world-economy" is key to understanding the development of a world-economy (p. 233). The relative position of one area versus another may change over time but the dynamics of the core and periphery relationship will hold. Out of this process there is a strong pattern about the strength of states; states in the core are strong and conversely states in the periphery are weak. The position that states have with each other is important since it can provide insight into the direction of the world-economy. He points out, which areas play what roles is in many ways accidental but what is necessary for a core state is that the state machinery be far stronger than in others (Wallerstein, 1974). If we substitute corporate power for state power a corollary between the strength of health care systems as they are emerging under the globalization pressures can be drawn. What this means is that the medical tourism providers, the large transnational health care corporations, and health insurance providers represent a newly defined portion of the "core" and will define the terms of the expansion of global health care. These new stake holders have the power and "machinery" to continue to expand into the periphery of newly developed medical care markets in a continuous drive for capital accumulation. Given the huge revenues generated by medical tourism, Wallerstein's analysis fits very well in terms of the ability of capital accumulation to break down national boundaries.

Yet, world-systems theory may not adequately explain the shifting contours of health care as a result of technology that means demographic shifts within new medical developments are putting new pressures on the medical infrastructure. Further, there are exogenous factors, such as the aging of baby boomers, that affect the ability of employers, states, and the Federal government to provide healthcare (Mutchnick et al., 2005; Turner, 2007). Certainly the critique can be made of world-systems theory does not adequately explain cultural globalism but explains it as a consequence of global economic forces. However, this critique cannot be applied at this point to an analysis of the globalization of health care using world-systems theory since there is only fragmented evidence of a global medical culture. Certainly there are pressures to standardize treatment for specific illnesses and this may result in a global medical culture in which case a reassessment of the usefulness of world-systems theory will need to be made.

Most, if not all, of the health care restructuring in recent years has been due to the economic role of health care in the economy of the countries seeking to control the amount spent on health care (Björkman & Altenstetter, 1997, p. 2). Medical tourism sits at the growing intersections of technology, economy, cultural, and other global relations and will play a significant role in shaping the future of medical care globally and locally. The notion of globalization has become one of the defining theoretical frameworks within sociology in recent decades despite the lack of consensus about a single definition of globalization. This points to a powerful need to grasp, explain, and perhaps predict the rapid shifts in social patterns and the reordering of economic, social, political, cultural global trends. This is equally true for the new patterns that will emerge as a result of medical tourism.

NOTES

1. The topic of the globalization of medicine and healthcare is much broader than the discussion in this paper and includes the globalization of medical education, movement of health care workers from one area to another, and the outsourcing of medical services like transcription and diagnostics.

2. Hereafter referred to as Hearings.

3. This does not imply that this is the best definition nor does it imply that this is the only definition of globalization. This is merely a definition that is readily available and understandable within the context of some of the analysis of these issues.

4. While it may be argued that the paraphrase is inappropriate, I none the less feel it captures the spirit of the point that Wallerstein was trying to make with regard to the expansion of a particular economic and social structure.

5. The definitions of the "core" sites of economic strength are covered in greater detail in Wallerstein's analysis. However, I believe that extending the definitions to the US medical establishment is appropriate and within the framework of the World System Analysis Wallerstein developed.

REFERENCES

Björkman, J., & Altenstetter, C. (1997). Executive summary and emerging themes. In: J. Björkman & C. Altenstetter (Eds), *Health policy reform, national variations and globalization*. New York, NY: St. Martin Press Inc.

Blue Shield of California. Access Baja Blue Shield. (2008). Accessed January 19, 2008. (https://www.blueshieldca.com/producer/largegroups/products/health/baja/).

Blumenthal, D. (2006) Employer-sponsored health insurance in the United States: Origins and Implications. *New England Journal of Medicine*, *355*(1), 82–88.

Burbach, R. (2001). *Globalization and postmodern politics from Zapatistas to high-tech Robber Barons*. Ann Arbor: University of Michigan Press.

Duffy, D. M. (1997). State, economy, and civil society interdependency: Lessons from the Polish health systems. In: J. Björkman & C. Altenstetter (Eds), *Health policy reform, national variations and globalization*. New York, NY: St. Martin's Press Inc.

El Taguri, A. (2007). Medical tourism and the Libyan national health services. *Libyan Journal of Medicine*, *2*, 1–4.

Fineberg, H. V. (1995). Crossing boundaries. In: P. Freeman, O. Gómez-Dantés & J. Frenk (Eds), *Health systems in an era of globalization: Challenges and opportunities, a conference summary*. Washington, DC: Board on International Health, Institute of Medicine.

Fuchs, V. R., & Ezekiel, J. E. (2005). Health care reform: Why? What? When? *Health Affairs*, *24*(6), 1399–1414.

Gabel, J., Claxton, G., Gil, I., Pickreign, J., Whitmore, H., Finder, B., Hawkins, S., & Rowland, D. (2005). Health benefits in 2005: Premium increases slow down, coverage continues to erode. *Health Affairs*, *24*, 1273–1280.

Giddens, A. (1990). *The consequences of modernity: Self and society in the late modern age*. Cambridge: Polity.

Gómez-Dantés, O., & Frenk, J. (1995). NAFTA and health services: Initial data. In: P. Freeman, O. Gómez-Dantés & J. Frenk (Eds), *Health systems in an era of globalization: Challenges and opportunities a conference summary*. Washington, DC: Board on International Health, Institute of Medicine.

Kher, U. (2006). Outsourcing your heart. *Time Magazine* (May 29), 44–47.

Maciel, M. L. (2003). Knowledge production as a Factor in World Polarization. In: W. A. Dunaway (Ed.), Emerging Issues in the 21st Century World-System (Contributions in Economics and Economic History, No. 230) Political Economy of the World-System Conference 2001. Praeger Publishers: CT.

MacIntosh, C. (2004). Medical tourism: need surgery will travel. CBSNews Online www.cbc.ca/news/background/healthcare/medicaltourism2.html. Accessed on February 12, 2008.

Milstein, A., & Smith, M. (2007). Will the surgical world become flat? *Health Affairs, 26*(1), 137–141.

Mutchnick, I., Stern, D. T., & Moyer, C. A. (2005). Trading health services across borders: GATS, markets, and caveats. *Health Affairs* (Web exclusive), 10.1377/hlthaff.w5.42. Posting date: January 25, 2005 by Project HOPE (http://content.healthaffairs.org/cgi/content/abstract/hlthaff.w5.42), accessed November 28, 2007.

Robertson, R. (1992). *Globalization: Social theory and global culture*. London: Sage.

Rodrik, D. (1997). *Has globalization gone too far?* Washington, DC: Institute for International Economics.

Rodwin, V. G. (1997). The rise of managed care in the United States: Lessons for French health policy. In: J. Björkman & C. Altenstetter (Eds), *Health policy reform, national variations and globalization*. New York, NY: St. Martin Press Inc.

Sinha, A. (2000). An overview of telemedicine: The virtual gaze of health care in the next century. *Medical Anthropology Quarterly*, New Series, *14*(3), 291–309.

Skarbinski, J., Walker, H. K., Laurence, C. B., Kobaladze, A., Kirtava, Z., & Raffin, T. A. (2002). The burden of out-of-pocket payments for health care in Tbilisi, Republic of Georgia. *JAMA*, *287*, 1043–1049.

Smith, R. D. (2004). Foreign direct investment and trade in health services: A review of the literature. *Social Science and Medicine, 59*, 2313–2323.

Starr, P. (1984). *The social transformation of American medicine: The rise of a sovereign profession and the making of a vast industry*. New York, NY: Basic Books.

Turner, L. (2007) First world health care at third world prices: Globalization, bioethics, and medical tourism *Biosocieties 2*, 303–325.

United States, Department of Commerce, Commercial Service, accessed August 4, 2008. (http://www.buyusa.gov/asianow/pmedical.html).

United States Senate Special Committee on Aging. (2006). "The globalization of health care: Can medical tourism reduce health care costs?" Senate Hearing, June 27, 2006. 109th Congress, Second Session. Washington: Government Printing Office.

Wallerstein, I. (1976 [1990]). *The modern world-system: Capitalist agriculture and the origins of the European world-economy in the sixteenth century*. New York, NY: Academic Press.